The PCG Development Guide

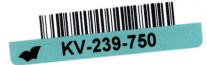

Edited by

Tim Wilson

Foreword by

Professor Mike Pringle

Radcliffe Medical Press

Radcliffe Medical Press Ltd
18 Marcham Road, Abingdon, Oxon OX14 1AA

British Library Cataloguing in Publication Data

A catalogue record for this book is available from the British Library.

ISBN 1 85775 332 1

Typeset by Advance Typesetting Ltd, Oxfordshire
Printed and bound by Hobbs the Printers, Totton, Hants

Contents

Foreword

In a career in general practice a doctor can expect an increasing number of major reorganisations. The advent of primary care groups is our latest such upheaval – and may be judged by history to be one of the most significant.

Primary care groups need to be seen in an historical context. The 1966 GP Charter laid this foundation stone for modern general practice with teams in adequate premises. The 1990 reforms were, arguably, intended to bring hospital consultants under control by making them sensitive to market pressures. Now in 1999 we see this refined. PCGs rid us of these inequalities of non-fundholding and fundholding, and the paper chase of the internal market. Yet, at the same time the pressure on hospital trusts will be intensified, with whole groups of practices demanding better services.

With hindsight it can be seen that the 1990 reforms contained a key flaw: the power shift to primary care was not accompanied by an increase in accountability. Fundholders were audited for their financial probity, not for their clinical effectiveness.

The design of PCGs puts accountability at the top of the agenda. The commissioning and delivery of primary care, the commissioning of secondary care, and the integration of social care will be assessed. Clinical governance, adoption of National Service Frameworks and NICE guidelines, changes in hospital services and collaboration with Social Services will all be measured and used in performance management.

This transition to a 'managed' service will be a bitter pill for many general practitioners and their staff – particularly, I suspect, practice managers used to the autonomy of fundholding. However, we have no real option. The loss of public confidence in the health service must be addressed and PCGs offer the mechanism for doing so while still retaining a strong professional involvement.

The reintroduction of doctors and other primary care clinicians into health service management, at a level above the practice, offers major challenges – for skills, co-operation, leadership and time. This challenge underlines the philosophy of this book.

All members of PCGs and their practices will need to develop a new range of expertise and this book offers practical help in defining and organising their expertise. This text is clear and informative. The style is accessible. The message is unequivocal – PCGs are an opportunity to maximise and a threat to control and minimise.

Professor Mike Pringle
April 1999

Preface

foreword

The introduction of primary care groups (PCGs) represents one of the biggest changes in primary care since the introduction of the NHS; this is a theme that is repeated throughout this book. Are PCGs good or bad? This is unimportant, they are here and everyone in primary care will be involved. As Alan Milburn, the former Minister of Health, was fond of saying, 'no change is not an option'. However, they not only offer great potential, but will also involve a considerable amount of work and a journey into uncharted territory.

The *PCG Development Guide* is a practical book designed to help those involved in PCGs. PCGs are likely to include many people with a considerable range of skills. However, they cannot be expected to know about everything covered in this book, particularly where new areas of work are involved. So who should read this book? First, board members, who are likely to find something in here of use to them. It will give them an understanding of the complexities involved in PCGs and how these may be overcome, either in areas of work they are involved in personally or in work their colleagues are doing. There are many others who will be involved in PCGs, directly or indirectly: health authority managers and personnel in social services, community and acute trusts, and Community Health Councils are but a few. They too should read this book.

The first six chapters are mainly concerned with the general management issues of PCGs. None are totally comprehensive; how could they be when entire textbooks are devoted to them? However, they give a clear picture of the issues involved and how PCGs may approach the different management functions. The authors are all people with experience or expertise in these fields.

Clinical governance is probably the most daunting task facing PCGs. For some it presents a major threat; however, it may be the last chance the medical profession has to pursue self-regulation. It may also offer the best chance for ensuring quality. Chapter 7 offers an excellent overview of clinical governance and how PCGs should be considering it.

The implication for primary care with the introduction of PCGs is great. GPs won many concessions and guarantees from the Minister of Health because of the possible changes. Chapter 8 offers a glimpse of how primary care and its development may change.

If PCGs are to succeed, they will have to make sure they are able to assess the needs of their population. The change in population size will mean a new perspective for PCGs. Further, they will have to make a meaningful contribution to Health Improvement Programmes, especially if they want their voice to be heard. This is considered in Chapter 9.

Although primary care and social services workers have collaborated in the past, this has been the exception rather than the rule. This should change with the introduction of PCGs, and will be new to many of those in PCGs, Chapter 10 will help you with joint working.

Public involvement is not an add-on, an annual general meeting will not do. Public involvement can mean many things and there are many models. It can be done in different ways for different purposes as described in Chapter 11.

There are many people who have valuable experience to offer PCGs. Nurses, who for the first time are involved in healthcare planning at this level, have many skills to offer. Fundholders and commissioning GPs have often been at opposite ends of the spectrum; however, they both have a lot to offer and to ignore the experience of one group would be a waste. Chapter 12 discusses this important issue.

There have been a number of models of primary care commissioning. The final chapter in this book gives some examples of what can be achieved, often very simply. PCGs may want to emulate some of these ideas.

In summary, after reading this book, you will have a clear view of what PCGs have to offer and what they will have to do to fulfil their potential.

Tim Wilson
April 1999

List of contributors

Fran Butler
Senior Project Officer
PCG Resource Unit

Professor Linda Challis
School of Healthcare
Oxford Brookes University

John Derry
Chair
Oxfordshire MAAG

Michael Dixon
Chair
NHS Alliance

Bruce Donn
Director
Bruce Donn Consulting Ltd
Toot Baldon, Oxford

Lorna Hipkin
Freelance Management Consultant
Chipping Norton, Oxon

Paul Johnstone
Public Health Consultant
Berkshire Health

Barbara Noakes
Primary Care Workforce Planning Officer
Public Health Resource Unit
Oxford

John Rawlinson
General Practitioner
Berkshire

Elaine Richardson
Human Resources Development Specialist
Bedfordshire Health Authority
Luton

David Rowson
Communications Manager
Berkshire Health Authority

Peter Smith
General Practitioner
Kingston-upon-Thames

Mary Wicks
Practice Manager
Wallingford Medical Centre

Tim Wilson
GP Director
PCG Resource Unit

Andrea Young
Director of Development
Oxfordshire Health Authority

Acknowledgements

Many thanks to all the authors, who worked so hard to produce their excellent chapters in such a short time. Thanks also to Sylvia Collins, in the Public Health Resource Unit, and my wife, for their support. Finally, thank you to Professor Ruth Chambers, who encouraged me to edit this book.

CHAPTER ONE

Management

Elaine Richardson

Primary care groups (PCGs) face a massive agenda over the next few years. Not only do they have to achieve the functions and tasks laid out in the White Paper[1] and Health Service Circular (HSC) 1998/139,[2] they also need to develop as organisations. So at the very time when a PCG is starting to develop its infrastructure it is required to produce concrete outputs to very tight timescales. Good management in PCGs will be essential if they are to successfully achieve all the tasks without burning out those involved. However, developing good management is not easy.

What is management?

Defining management is itself a difficult task. Charles Handy describes it as a creative and political process rather than a precise science,[3] and Robert Heller dares to suggest that it does not exist and, being amorphous and shifting, can be defined in almost any way.[4] This may explain why what many people have done is to describe the role or principles of management rather than define management itself. The various role descriptions are all about enabling others to deliver, such as Tony Ball's 'to remove the blocks to others' performance'.[5] Ball also suggests that one of the problems with management today is that rather than concentrating on that role, managers have become 'enmeshed in a mountainous list of duties'. This is certainly true in many areas of the NHS, where a manager is very much seen as a doer. Rosemary Stewart sets out some useful role distinctions in *Leading in the NHS: a practical guide*.[6] She describes leadership as discovering the route ahead, encouraging and inspiring others to follow; management as implementing the vision through the discipline of objectives, targets and reviews; and administration as carrying out the policies and being publicly accountable for doing so. She sums the roles up as follows:

- Administrators confirm in writing.

- Managers direct.
- Leaders point the way: identify and symbolise what is important.

All three roles are important and will be needed in PCGs, but before management roles are defined and structures set up, PCGs need to think through the organisation they wish to create.

When working under the sorts of pressures that PCGs are experiencing, it is easy to fall into the trap of sticking with what you know. Unfortunately this tends to result in structures and systems that people are used to, rather than the development of those that will deliver what is needed long term. One of the most useful things a shadow PCG can do, is give itself the space to think through the following three questions:

- What do we want to be?
- Where are we now?
- How will we get there?

It does not have to be a long drawn out exercise and some of the thinking may well have already been started, if not completed. But only when the first two have been explored can the appropriate management structures and systems really be developed. If time and energy are not invested in thinking these things through, PCGs may find themselves with teams that are designed for a different game to the one they really want to play.

One of the biggest problems in trying to write on management in a way that a PCG may find useful, is that there are likely to be as many different approaches to managing PCGs as there are PCGs. Even HSC 1998/139 acknowledges that a PCG should develop in a way that is 'appropriate to local circumstances in which it operates'.[7] This chapter therefore tries to set out some pointers rather than give answers, but be aware it may well raise even more questions for those involved in developing PCGs.

Where do we want to be?

When asking this question you need to think of both the immediate and longer term. The danger is to allow the timescales in the guidance to focus the PCG too closely on the immediate deliverables, especially when no one is really clear what the long term will hold. Developing a vision of where the PCG wants to be is not just around the level at which it wants to operate but also about how the individuals within it want to work. Huczynski and Buchanan[8] suggest that only the individuals within organisations have goals, not the organisations themselves, and that in some cases the goals of individuals may be different from the collective purpose of the organised activity. This provides an interesting challenge for PCGs, because while they exist, they are not strictly organisations in their own right. They could be described as virtual organisations rather than real ones, being made up of a network of organisations that are both independent and accountable to one another by virtue of the fact they hold collective responsibility.

While the context for the vision of a PCG is to a large extent dictated by the government and possibly by their health authority, PCGs can decide how they shape the vision. The main focus for PCGs will be around patient care and it is worth remembering that both managers and clinicians have a goal of effective patient care, they just come at it from different perspectives. It is unrealistic to expect non-clinicians to be able to make decisions on resources that will please clinicians, just as it is unrealistic to expect all clinicians to want to spend their time in detailed management tasks rather than working with patients. The art will be getting the correct balance to achieve a successful PCG, for example freeing up GP and nurse time so they can take a lead on service development, and setting up management structures that support them in that process.

Where are we now?

Charles Handy warns that 'many of the ills of organisations stem from imposing an inappropriate structure on a particular culture, or from expecting a particular culture to thrive in an inappropriate climate'.[9] So it is useful to think through the culture of PCGs and the climate in which they are operating.

The culture of organisation is in itself a complex subject and there are many books and papers about it. However, PCGs may find Charles Handy's descriptions of four main types of culture[10] a useful framework, as they highlight some of the key issues PCGs and the stakeholder organisations will face when developing management structures.

Power

This is very much a patriarchal culture where the central individual holds the power and influence. This power tends to be resource- and personnel-based and becomes less important to people the further away they are from the centre. The organisation functions through empathy, trust and affinity with face-to-face communication and little bureaucracy. This enables quick decisions to be made but the organisation is very dependent on those at the centre and cannot survive if it grows too big.

Role

This is the 'typical' organisation with clearly defined job roles, rules and procedures, and lots of bureaucracy. Position power is the main source of power, with the procedures and rules having the greatest influence. A board or management group heads up a role organisation but its strength lies in its functions or specialities. So survival relies on and encourages stability and predictability. Role organisations often try to ignore change and tend to develop cross-functional links as a way of strengthening the organisation if it seems in danger of collapse.

Task

A task organisation uses expert power with much of the power and influence lying at certain points like the interstices of the net. Control is difficult for top management, as it can only be strategic and not day-to-day. Sections are largely self-contained, as their main concern is developing solutions to the problem but they work within an overall strategy. Mutual respect and a desire to help are common, with team objectives being stronger than personal ones. A true task organisation can work quickly, as each group holds all the decision-making powers it needs to get on with the job, so it remains flexible. However, it actually needs variety to survive. It can be an expensive organisation as it is staffed by experts and it needs plenty of resources or groups will find themselves competing.

Person

This culture differs from the other three, as in them the individual serves the organisation, but in the person culture the organisation serves the individuals within it. Such organisations generally involve professionals, as they enable freedom and personal identity while providing support, flexibility and bargaining power. Personal power reigns, as influence and power lies with each individual. Management is therefore by consent rather than delegated authority and is usually seen as a chore. Such organisations tend to have to remain small and often they develop their own identity and start to impose on the individuals so becoming one of the other three cultures.

When looking at the stakeholder organisations involved in PCGs the different cultures can be seen. Most GP practices are person cultures with some having developed into task, role or power, whereas health authorities, trusts and local government are notoriously role or possibly task cultures. PCGs will need to acknowledge these variations and find a way of working with them. The structure and lines of accountability set out in the guidance point to a role culture, with PCGs having boards that are subcommittees of the health authority. However, it is possible to develop a way of working that retains this structure while allowing a task culture, but it will be difficult to retain a strong person culture.

   With regard to the climate, an analogy used by Rosabeth Moss Kanter to describe the ever-changing climate in which businesses are trying to operate seems equally appropriate to the NHS.[11] The analogy is the croquet game in *Alice in Wonderland* where Alice is trying to use a mallet that lifts its head, to hit a hedgehog ball that unrolls, moves to somewhere else and rolls up again, towards hoops that move when the queen orders them to. Not surprisingly Alice found it very difficult to compete, as the various organisations involved in PCGs are finding it. PCGs are not completely masters of their own destiny so it is important to recognise the 'givens' and work with them rather than expending energy trying to change them at the beginning. This is not to say PCGs should just accept everything without challenge, but it is easier to influence the direction of a vehicle that is moving than one that is bogged down in the mud.

The changing climate is not a new issue for PCG stakeholders. GPs and the health authority in particular have experienced major changes through the introduction of the internal market and fundholding. Social services have been through similar changes and have their own White Paper to deal with. The effects of these changes cannot be ignored, as they will impact on how PCG stakeholders perceive and trust each other. Acknowledging that everyone brings with them baggage from the past and trying to work with that will be important for PCGs, especially where relationships that were previously managerial are now partnerships.

Another issue that needs to be considered is the fact that the GPs and nurses who are the backbone of the PCG already have jobs working directly with patients. Workload is already increasing due to patient demand and adding another layer of roles and responsibility will add to the stress on both the individuals and the system. If they are to survive, PCGs and the people in them will have to embrace the adage that it is necessary to work 'smarter not harder'.

How will we get there?

HSC 1998/139[2] laid down some of the fundamentals, such as board composition, the accountability structure and the key responsibilities of the PCG Chair, Chief Officer and stakeholders. Because of the tight timescales, board members will have been elected/ selected possibly using role specifications developed by the health authority. It is likely that many of these role specifications will have been written from a structural perspective rather than a functional one, as there has been little time to ask the PCG the 'Where do you want to be?' question. PCGs must decide how they wish to use any role specifications both to ensure flexibility and to take ownership of the positions. Role specifications can be very useful but they can also reinforce an inflexible role culture that may well not be appropriate in a PCG.

In the light of the guidance, it is not surprising that most of the initial effort will have been focused on the Board. While this will need to be addressed in the longer term, by concentrating on the Board and considering its functions, the other management needs of the PCG will become clearer.

The role of the Board

As a subcommittee of a health authority the PCG board may find itself based on the model of a health authority board, so for this reason it is useful to consider the typical NHS board. The structure is based on the model used in business, that is, chair, executive directors including the chief executive, and non-executive directors, but it operates under a different corporate governance system. In the NHS, corporate governance involves accountability, probity and openness. The National Association of Health Authorities and Trusts (NAHAT)[12] sets out six key functions that NHS boards are accountable for:

- formulating a strategy for operation within the policies and priorities of the NHS
- overseeing the administration of the strategy
- ensuring a high standard of financial stewardship
- ensuring a high standard of corporate governance and personal behaviour
- appointing senior executives and evaluating their performance
- maintaining an effective dialogue with the local community.

PCG boards will need to balance all these functions to avoid the danger highlighted by Sir John Harvey Jones[13] of boards allowing their 'legal' responsibility to take them over at the expense of strategy review and effective staff recruitment. Boards must ensure they are clear about the management structure they want, the sort of people they wish to appoint and who will be involved in the selection process. These last two are particularly important, as the Chief Officer is likely to be an employee of the health authority.

While all the directors on the Board are equal in status and hold corporate responsibility for any work carried out in their name, the board members hold different roles.

- Chair: leader of the Board, so responsible and accountable for its behaviour and decisions.
- Chief Executive: responsible to Chair for the effective management of the organisation.
- Executive directors: responsible to the Chief Executive for the management of the organisation.
- Non-executive directors: responsible for setting direction, developing strategy and monitoring progress.

Whether PCG boards need an executive/non-executive split is debatable, not least because not all of the organisations involved in PCGs will have a representative on the Board. PCG board members would be better operating as non-executive directors developing sub-structures that will enable the PCG to manage the business in order to deliver against the strategies. This should help prevent a problem Bob Garratt identifies for boards where directors retain their operational role rather than starting to spend their time thinking and reflecting in order to give direction.[14] Effective delegation is the key to gaining the time to look holistically across the whole organisation.

Delegation is also essential, as while the Board is accountable, the wrecking power lies with individuals. HSC 1998/139[2] makes it very clear that GPs retain the right to refer and prescribe as they see fit. Having the discussions and making the decisions at board level is unlikely to change the behaviour of all individuals. The fact the Board can co-opt as necessary is one way of trying to gain ownership, however, delegation to subgroups is likely to be a better way. The Board can then take more responsibility for the process by which subgroups arrive at decisions rather than getting bogged down in the decision itself.

Effective delegation can be achieved by following a four-step process.

1   **Be clear what is being delegated** – People are more motivated if they can take responsibility for the whole rather than bits. Delegating the whole project also makes it easier to see its context, importance and impact, and leaves scope for freedom. Likewise it is better to delegate in terms of outcomes or results rather than process, as this enables those delegated to, to take the initiative. An important aspect of delegation to remember is that while the accountability remains with the Board, the responsibility and authority must be delegated as part of the project.

2   **Agree time frames, feedback mechanisms and controls** – Right from the start both the person delegating and the people being delegated to must agree deadlines, monitoring processes and feedback mechanisms. Unrealistic deadlines are demotivating and lack of deadlines tends to allow other work pressures to take priority. The monitoring process should provide support for those delegated to as well as reassuring the person delegating that they are not going to be held accountable for a disaster. It is not advisable to do spot checks outside of the agreed process as it implies a lack of confidence. Regular feedback is important as it will help the project stay on course and give the Board the necessary management information. The Board is also aware of any issues that are beyond the project group's control and if necessary can take the appropriate action.

3   **Check out understanding** – The most dangerous aspect of any delegation process is to assume that the understanding of the project is the same for everyone. The person delegating must check that those who are being delegated to understand precisely what is expected of them. This is particularly important with regard to their authority, as they need to be clear as to whether they can proceed without prior approval, proceed but keep informed or whether they need to obtain approval first. Budgetary issues in particular may fall into the last category.

4   **Let go** – For many this is the hardest part but, provided the other steps have been followed, the Board should be confident enough to allow the project group to get on with it. If the group comes back for support it is advisable to adopt the approach of helping them to answer their own questions rather than giving answers, and if things do go wrong let the group correct their mistakes, having given the necessary support first.

Effective delegation requires the investment of time, especially at the beginning, but the return on that investment includes greater ownership, increased motivation, individual development and succession planning as well as achieving the project outcome.

Common pitfalls in the use of resources

Management by committee or group is common in organisations and works on the basis that group decisions are better than individual ones. This is likely to be the case in PCGs, as the groups will be composed of a mixture of people bringing very different perspectives. However, one of the most common problems with management groups is that they are resource expensive. The most valuable resources PCGs have are the people involved in them. The art of good management for PCGs will therefore lie with using their people resources effectively and efficiently. There are five common ways of wasting resources that PCGs will do well to avoid:

- using the wrong resources
- duplication
- failing to end
- lack of synergy in groups
- group-think.

Using the wrong resources

The nature of the work of the PCG in having to:

- develop and implement strategic and business plans for services
- provide information that enables sound financial management of the PCG budget
- deliver and report on governance and accountability
- ensure delivery on areas such as clinical governance
- promote personal and organisational development

will involve all three roles of leader, manager and administrator. PCGs would do well to ensure that the appropriate resource is used in each. Many organisations still frequently use managers to carry out work that an administrator would be better equipped to do and assume leaders are capable of carrying out management tasks. At best this results in inefficient use of resources and at worst ineffective use.

The Chief Officer needs to be a manager, leader or mixture of both, depending on the vision of the PCG and the skills and expertise it already has. If the vision is to change service delivery, clinicians will need to take the lead with the Chief Officer developing the underpinning management systems and administrators doing the supporting work. If the vision is to build the PCG as an organisation in order to become a primary care trust, then a chief officer who can create a vision of a partnership organisation will be needed. As such, he or she will hold a 'general manager'-level post and will need other managers as well as administrators to develop systems that will deliver the vision.

It is likely the Chair and the Chief Officer, while being in a line management role, will share some of the leadership of the PCG, especially as the time commitment of the Chair is likely to be more limited than that of the Chief Officer. To do this effectively they will need to develop a close productive working relationship agreeing strategies and the roles they will play in situations.

HSC 1998/139[2] puts much of the responsibility for PCGs on to health authorities and confirms that they will be performance managed on the development and operation of the PCGs in their area. A relationship based on interdependency would therefore be a wise one, with PCGs actively seeking help and support from the health authority and keeping them informed of what they are doing while at the same time demonstrating their ability. Understandably a health authority will not want to delegate responsibilities to a PCG unless it is certain it can discharge them properly. So PCGs and health authorities must discuss the issue of the delegation of responsibilities and reach an agreed decision. Like any good delegation process, a relationship that gives PCGs the opportunity to check out their understanding or actions before actually committing themselves is more likely to result in success.

Within PCGs individuals and the Board must recognise their limitations and work with others as and when necessary. This help may come from within the PCG or from outside, such as from the health authority. For example, health authority managers are used to working with the bureaucracy of the NHS and their help will be valuable when trying to find extra funding or produce documents that will satisfy the system. At board level, co-opting a health authority finance lead may be a very prudent move as the budget is ultimately the responsibility of the health authority. PCGs should find that their health authority is a useful ally, especially in the shadow period.

Duplication

Duplication is a common waste of resources. At board level it often occurs where executive committees are set up, as these generally result in matters already discussed at length by the Executive being rediscussed by the Board. While PCGs may not have executive committees, the subgroups that report to the Board may suffer the same duplication. There is nothing wrong in having items on the agenda of a board meeting that are for notification or to gain opinions rather than for real discussion and decision making. But if the balance is wrong and board members feel their advice is not being sought or acted on, the Board will become impoverished. Using board members in subgroups may help prevent this.

Duplication may occur not only within the PCG, but it may also arise between the PCG and the health authority, especially when PCGs are keen to get on with things. A considerable amount of skill, knowledge and experience which will be of tremendous use to PCGs is held within the health authority. And learning to utilise it will be a major advantage to a PCG. Where health authorities are happy to continue to do some of the work that could be taken on by PCGs it may be best to let them, especially if by taking it on themselves a PCG is duplicating work, e.g. contracting or developing certain strategies. In other areas the health authority may already have strategies and systems that can be tweaked to meet the needs of the PCG, for example public involvement. It may also be appropriate for PCGs to continue to use some of the health authority expertise in the longer term, for example public health, finance and IM&T rather than for PCGs to try to develop it in-house.

Sharing resources will enable more effective solutions to be found for some of the problems that exist for the constituent organisations. For example, a pharmacist working for a PCG will be able to undertake different projects for a number of practices, so giving each practice direct help in one area while at the same time enabling the practice to learn from the projects being carried out in the other practices. Developing expertise in one or two individuals for the benefit of all of the stakeholder organisations will enable a better return on investment than developing one per organisation, e.g. public involvement skills or technical information technology (IT) skills. Cost-effectiveness will probably drive some of the collegiate working across PCGs. However, this will need to be weighed against the need for local variations. Joint working brings its own set of problems, but these usually arise because the joint working is not properly integrated in the role of the individual and so conflicts of agenda arise. By adopting a consultant/contractor-type relationship, where the individual has a specific role or service to deliver and the employment lines are purely there to protect the individual, some of these difficulties are overcome.

Failing to end

Some organisations set up groups but forget to give them a clear goal, which once achieved will mean the group is no longer needed. PCGs will need to put a lot of effort into a variety of areas in the early stages at a pace that will not be sustainable in the longer term. Groups need to be clear on what they are being asked to achieve so they can plan their work around it. Then when the goal is achieved the group can celebrate and disband. Some work may well spawn another group, but it should be seen as a new group with a new objective rather than a continuation of the original.

When a project contains phases that need different expertise, don't fall into the trap of involving everyone to the same extent all the way through. The first meeting may involve everyone to set the scene and agree the plan, but then expertise should be brought in to each phase as appropriate.

By setting clear objectives for its working groups, a PCG will be able to utilise its resources more effectively and prevent people feeling they are meeting for the sake of it. This should in turn keep motivation high.

All three of the pitfalls described above can be avoided by adopting good project planning and project management techniques at all levels within the PCG.

Good project planning involves seven stages:

1   identifying the end goal and its standard
2   identifying the tasks and milestones along the way
3   sequencing the tasks and milestones and noting any dependencies
4   identifying time frames and deadlines
5   identifying resources (e.g. people, financial, equipment) and any constraints
6   gaining commitment from individuals and allocating resources
7   agreeing how progress will be monitored and the project reviewed.

Stages 5 and 6 will impact on each other, with some deadlines preventing the involvement of certain people due to the fact they are unavailable or work part time. A decision has to be reached as to which factor has priority, i.e. is the deadline imposed and non-negotiable or is the involvement of a particular individual more important than the deadline? There are tools available to help project planning, such as Gantt charts. These give a graphical representation of the tasks involved in a project and help ensure that tasks are scheduled in a logical way, taking account of the fact that some may be dependent on the completion of others. The resources available to carry out the tasks can also be plotted on the chart to help set realistic time frames, e.g. a five-day task involving one particular person who works three days a week cannot be completed in a calendar week. Good project management then involves implementing stage 7.

The submission of good project plans to PCG boards will give them the confidence to retain a hands-off approach, thereby leaving the project team to get on with it. The Board should remain informed through the project management process, which will include submitting regular progress reports. In this way the Board need only get involved when their help is needed.

Unfortunately the final two pitfalls can occur even when projects are well-planned and properly managed as they arise from working within groups.

Lack of synergy in groups

Social processes mean that individuals within groups will often compromise their views, the result being that extreme views are moderated and compromise is reached to the detriment of the decision-making process. Jay Hall concluded that effective groups actively look for points of disagreement and consequently encourage conflict in the early stages of a discussion.[15] PCG board meetings in particular may suffer from a lack of synergy, as they are open and this may well have a restraining influence on the members. One way around this would be for the Chair to open meetings by explaining how the decision process will operate thereby 'giving permission' for challenge and conflict. All groups operating within PCGs should strive to achieve consensus and not lose synergy by fundamentally accepting that differences of opinion are natural and should be encouraged. In this way a greater range of information is likely to be considered, resulting in decisions that are acceptable to all and greater than that of any one individual.

Key behaviours to avoid are arguing for your own point of view while not listening to others, changing opinions to appease others, reaching decisions too quickly, majority voting and bargaining.

Group-think

Group-think, while similar to lack of synergy in that disagreement is discouraged, can have an even greater detrimental effect. Irving Janis cites it as a reason for a number of disasters in American foreign policy and describes it as 'the psychological drive for consensus at any cost that suppresses dissent and appraisal of alternatives in cohesive decision making groups'.[16] Symptoms of group-think include the group closing ranks with members, so not discussing any unease outside the group. Dissent may even be suppressed within the group, with contrary evidence being explained away or negative stereotypes being associated with those that raise it. One of the greatest worries for PCGs will be if groups display the symptom of invulnerability and take risks without realising the dangers.

PCGs can prevent group-think if:

- leaders of groups actively encourage open expression of doubt and welcome criticism of opinions, possibly assigning someone the role of devil's advocate
- expertise is not used selectively and 'higher status' members are invited to offer their opinions last
- conflicting evidence and alternatives are actively sought not hidden or immediately discounted
- reactions and recommendations are sought from outside the group or from a duplicate group
- the group periodically divides into subgroups.

As PCGs are likely to bring together new groups that are not too used to each other, group-think will not be an immediate problem. But it would be sensible to adopt the preventive measures from the beginning to avoid the need for a cure later on.

Perfect management of a PCG

While this is an interesting ideal and impossible dream, it is worth striving for and investing in. The success of a PCG will depend on its ability to operate in an environment of partnership and co-operation, that is to involve its constituent individuals and work with the health authority to develop arrangements and systems that enable independence in carrying out the day-to-day business. PCGs will need an influencing and empowering management system that creates an environment that frees up individuals to do the work that effects the PCG.

It is also worth remembering that PCGs are evolving organisations and as such need to retain flexibility in order to be able to continue to grow and succeed in the changing climate of the NHS. The greatest challenge for PCG management teams will be how to create an environment of learning.

References

1   Department of Health (1997) *The New NHS: modern, dependable*. Stationery Office, London.

2   NHS Executive (1998) *Developing Primary Care Groups*. HSC 1998/139. NHSE, London.

3   Handy C (1993) *Understanding Organisations* (4e). Penguin Books, Harmondsworth.

4   Heller R (1990) *The Making Of Managers.* Penguin Books, Harmondsworth, p 12.

5   Ball T (1994) Blocks to better management. *Management Development Review.* **7**(4): 14–15.

6   Stewart R (1996) *Leading in the NHS: a practical guide* (2e). Macmillan Press, Basingstoke, pp 3–5.

7   NHS Executive (1998) *Developing Primary Care Groups.* HSC 1998/139, p 3.

8   Huczynski A, Buchanan D (1991) *Organization Behaviour: an introductory text* (2e). Prentice Hall, New York, p 10.

9   Handy C (1993) *Understanding Organisations* (4e). Penguin Books, Harmondsworth, p 180.

10 Handy C (1991) *Gods of Management* (3e). Business Books, London.

11 Moss Kanter R (1994) *When Giants Learn to Dance.* Routledge, London, p 19.

12 Wall A (1993) *Healthy NHS Boards.* NAHAT, Birmingham.

13 Harvey-Jones J (1994) *Making It Happen,* Harper Collins, London, p 216.

14 Garratt B (1995) *Learning To Lead.* Harper Collins, London.

15 Huczynski A, Buchanan D (1991) *Organization Behaviour: an introductory text* (2e). Prentice Hall, New York, p 248.

16 Huczynski A, Buchanan D (1991) *Organization Behaviour: an introductory text* (2e). Prentice Hall, New York, pp 250–1.

CHAPTER TWO

Human resource and workforce planning issues

Barbara Noakes

The Government will work with the one million staff in the NHS to build a modern and dependable health service.

The New NHS: modern, dependable (December 1997)

Introduction

With the publication of the White Paper '*The New NHS: modern, dependable*'[1] in December 1997, the Government heralded a major period of organisational change in the NHS with the declared aim of improving quality and efficiency. A significant element of this programme of change is the development of primary care groups (PCGs).

Key to the successful development of these PCGs will be their ability to achieve a radical review and overhaul of the current organisational culture and working practices within primary care. In doing so they will need to develop a new joint working culture. This will mean moving from a system which involves small organisations led by GPs, either in partnerships or single-handed, generally caring for populations of between 2000 and 26 000 people, to the concept of those same practices working co-operatively within a much larger organisation – the PCG. The PCG will plan and deliver services of high quality and efficiency to much larger populations of between 50 000 and 250 000 people.

This chapter aims to consider those human resource issues that the PCGs will need to address to achieve their development as primary care trusts and to evolve as successful, efficient organisations. Bringing together what were previously independent and separate employers and asking them to review how the human resources they employ are used, may result in potential conflict and difficult choices having to be made. The experiences of GPs who have established out-of-hours co-operatives and those who have been involved in locality commissioning auger well, however, and have proved that it is possible to work together co-operatively and towards common goals.

Why bother?

Why do PCGs need to be concerned about human resource issues? Put simply, the answer is that PCGs cannot afford *not* to be concerned with the human resources they employ. First, it is a widely recognised and often-stated truism that an organisation's human resources are its most valuable asset and that without the talents, skills and dedication of the staff they employ, organisations cannot operate effectively. Second, while being its most valuable asset, an organisation's human resources are also its most expensive one. PCGs will need to look at themselves critically if they are to adequately assess whether they have the required human resources and whether they are being deployed and used effectively and efficiently.

Other reasons for needing to address the human resources agenda include the need to develop a consistent PCG-wide approach to:

- cope with the period of organisational change consequent upon the development of PCGs
- meet the requirements of employment legislation in the development of personnel policies and procedures
- meet the staff training and development requirements of government initiatives, such as those relating to public health and health promotion, clinical governance and the quality framework, and working in partnership with other organisations
- assist employees with dealing with the increasing expectations of the public as to what the service can offer.

Dealing with all of these will require the constituent employers to co-operate and work together to an extent that was unheard of before.

The recently published national human resources strategy for the NHS, *Working Together: securing a quality workforce for the NHS*,[2] details a number of key strategic aims and target areas to be achieved throughout the health service on a national and local basis. These are:

- To ensure a quality workforce, in the right numbers, with the right skills and diversity, organised in the right way, to deliver the Government's service objectives for health and social care.

- To demonstrate that steps are being taken to improve the quality of working life for staff.
- To address management capacity and capability to deliver this agenda and programme of change.

Primary care has in the past been seen as outside the mainstream of the NHS in terms of employment issues. Significantly the new human resources strategy makes it clear that PCGs as employers will be expected to comply with the requirements laid down in the framework document and meet the national minimum standards on human resource issues outlined by the NHS Executive. This crucial change in approach is very much a part of the concept of viewing all primary care employers as a member of what is now termed the 'NHS family'.

This change in approach obviously represents a significant organisational development challenge for PCGs and their constituent employers and they must consider how they will deal with it. In doing so they will need to develop a human resource strategy which not only incorporates meeting the national human resource standards as part of the long-term objectives of the new organisation, but also aims to deal with organisational development needs in the short term.

A human resource strategy for a PCG

Human resource strategies are about making business strategies work. The human resources strategy for the PCG must aim to create a unified working environment which will motivate, educate and develop people employed by a number of different employers, and maximise their contribution towards the achievement of the new organisation's objectives. (In this case the provision of the best quality healthcare to the local population.) It will therefore include the following key features:

- the organisation's 'vision' for the future
- an effective communications system
- a plan for achieving the optimum workforce
- a training and development plan
- employee relations agreements
- recruitment and selection
- staff health and welfare support.

These are explained in more detail below.

A 'vision' for the future

Fundamental to the change in the culture and working practices within primary care will be the need for the PCG to develop a 'vision' for the future that all staff, regardless of where they work, including those involved in the delivery of services, can relate to. All staff will need to know:

- What are the aims of the new organisation?
- What is it trying to achieve?
- What role do they as employees have in the achievement of the aims and how will they be supported in carrying it out?

Only when it reaches trust status will the PCG be able to employ staff directly. Recognising staff loyalties to their current organisation, the PCG Board must provide leadership and give both purpose and direction to harness the energy and commitment which already exists within primary healthcare teams. By developing and communicating to all employees – regardless of who their current employer is – a 'vision' which sets out the service goals and targets and how it is envisaged these will be achieved, employees will feel more comfortable with their role within the new organisation. To communicate the 'vision' is not enough however. The Board must consider how employees at all levels and locations will contribute to achieving the 'vision' and specify how individual development needs in particular will be assessed and met. This 'vision' will be fundamental to the maintenance of staff morale during the period of change and will enable staff to relate and contribute positively to changes being made.

Communications systems

It is widely recognised that the ability to communicate effectively is crucial to good management, particularly during periods of change, to ensure that staff are kept adequately informed, to reduce uncertainty and maintain morale. PCG boards will have to overcome the problems of staff not only employed by different organisations under the PCG umbrella but also based in a number of different geographical locations. If the cultural changes are to be implemented successfully, communication with staff at all levels and locations will have to remain high on the PCG Board agenda. The means of communication may vary according to the size and make-up of the PCG, but initiatives such as the establishment of regular newsletters and staff briefing sessions which provide accessible, consistent and unambiguous messages as well as the means to provide feedback are vital.

The individual counselling of staff affected by change will also be crucial to the future success of the organisation and in some cases external counselling and support may be necessary.

A plan for achieving the optimum workforce

Having agreed the 'vision' for the organisation and what it aims to achieve, the PCG will need to develop medium- and long-term plans for the delivery of service goals that are consistent with both national and local priorities for health.

At all levels of the NHS significant effort is put into predicting future demand and developing service plans to deal with the needs of the population. As they develop, PCGs will be no exception to this. It has to be recognised, however, that unless those service plans are integrated with a workforce plan to ensure that the right numbers of suitably trained staff are available where and when they are needed, the detailed service plans will simply not be achievable.

By linking the workforce and service needs it should be possible to plan over a 3–5-year period to:

- optimise the use of human resources and/or make them more flexible
- ensure that the short-term focus does not predominate and, by looking ahead, guarantee that the necessary expertise is available in the future given the extended training periods for a number of health professionals
- identify the areas where a shortage or excess of human resources is likely to occur in the future, or where there is an inefficient use of people
- highlight where there is a necessity to acquire and develop skills which otherwise may be short supply.

Using health visiting as a working example, it is possible to consider how an integrated service and workforce plan could be developed by the PCG as a trust responsible for employing the staff or working closely with the organisation from which services are commissioned.

Health visitors have traditionally specialised in health promotion and health surveillance, working mainly with mothers and young children but on occasion with all members of a family, including elderly people. It is recognised that the Government sees health visitors playing a key role in the successful delivery of its family policy initiatives. This is likely to result in an increased role for health visitors in the community, with greater involvement in the area of health needs assessment, health promotion and parental guidance. This will have a major impact on workloads at a time when there is a national shortage of health visitors and approximately 25% of those in post are approaching retirement age. The PCG must therefore plan ahead to ensure that it will be able to retain and attract sufficient staff to meet the needs of health visiting and where there are shortages of trained health visitors consider other options for meeting the service needs.

The ability to plan ahead is reliant upon the PCG having sufficient data available on the current workforce and the external labour market to enable trends and problems to be highlighted and to take account of these in making plans for the future. PCGs must develop an understanding of the workforce they employ and the labour markets within which they work and compete for skilled staff. They must recognise that there are different markets for different types of workers; normally they can look to the local labour market for part-time, lower-paid or less-skilled posts but may need to look further afield, nationally and perhaps internationally, to fill more senior professional posts.

What data are required?

The information required for workforce planning purposes can be divided into four main classifications. Examples of the information and their uses are given in the Appendix (p 25). The four main classifications are:

- data to give the historical perspective and highlight trends
- data to highlight current issues/problems
- data to inform future planning
- data on the external labour market.

In predicting demand, the PCG in our example must consider whether:

- the current establishment for health visitors is sufficient to meet existing service needs
- changes in the service will increase or decrease demand for qualified health visitors
- staff retiring will increase the numbers of vacant posts in the future
- funding is available to meet the additional costs if extra staff are required
- skill shortages locally and nationally have resulted in recruitment or retention difficulties
- a high staff turnover has caused problems.

Other questions to be considered include:

- Are there possibilities for part or all of the service to be streamlined across the PCG area?
- Do opportunities exist for the sharing of skills and workload with other professionals if demand and workload increases?
- Are there aspects of the job that could be carried out by less qualified but appropriately trained personnel?
- Are there any aspects of the job that could be redesigned /dropped?
- Could existing or anticipated recruitment and retention difficulties be alleviated by offering training, flexible working opportunities or other incentives to attract staff?
- Have the local education and training consortia been asked to amend their commissions for newly qualified staff or to support return to practice training in view of changes in demand and supply of health visitors?

Exploring these and other questions will assist the PCG in formulating a workforce plan to cope with the service needs. It will include a prediction of future staffing needs and a strategy to reduce adverse trends and promote positive changes.

The workforce plan and the data supporting it need to be regularly monitored and reviewed over time, however, if the PCGs are to continue to have the required capacity within their human resources to deliver the service requirements. By doing so it will be possible to anticipate and deal with any problems that arise.

An example of how such monitoring can be useful is in the consideration of staff turnover. Using the health visiting example again, the PCG Board may be concerned if the workforce data indicate that turnover for health visitors is high in comparison with the rest of the organisation. It is critical, however, that the causes of turnover are monitored, identified and fully understood. A certain level of turnover can be viewed as healthy because it can offer the opportunity of recruiting 'new blood' and fresh ideas into an organisation as well as providing career development opportunities for those staff who remain. However, if turnover is high for adverse reasons, it can affect the morale and motivation of the remaining staff, who may be overstressed as a result. In such cases action must be taken to eliminate those negative factors that are causing staff to leave. Similarly details of vacant posts and the length of time that posts are vacant can highlight particular recruitment problems and may indicate the need to consider alternative ways of filling a vacancy, possibly by using different types of staff or by trying a different approach to the recruitment problem. For example, it may be necessary to consider the introduction of more flexible employment practices, such as part-time working, job sharing, term-time only contracts or temporary employment, to attract new staff. It may also be necessary to consider offering return-to-work or update training to potential job applicants.

Workforce plans and supporting data can, if they are regularly monitored and adapted to suit changing circumstances, enable the PCG to have some control over something that is often seen as an unpredictable – the demand and supply of human resources. Changing circumstances and outside influences mean that supply and demand may never completely match, but by producing a plan and developing strategies to deal with shortfalls in supply, the PCG can make the problem more manageable.

Training and development

Chapter 3 discusses how PCGs identify and meet the training needs of their employees. It is important, however, that this exercise is seen as part of the overall human resource strategy and not separate from it. How people are developed is crucial to how they view an organisation and its commitment to them as individuals, and can be a key means of attracting or retaining staff, particularly during a period of change. Education levels and expectations continue to rise among employees, making them less willing to accept work that allows little opportunity for personal development and pride in their job. If individuals can see that their future development is interlinked with the success of the organisation and its achievement of its key service goals they are more likely to accept new forms of work organisation and successfully contribute to the organisation's enhanced performance.

It is therefore necessary to combine the 'vision' and goals of the organisation with the expectations and goals of the individual. This can usually be done through the use of personal development planning for all employees based on a system that regularly reviews and records an assessment of an employee's performance, potential and developmental needs linked to the overall objectives of the organisation. This process can be particularly important in developing teams with the right mix of skills and knowledge. It is also useful for assessing progress against service goals, looking back on what has been achieved, and agreeing objectives and development needs for the future against the goals and targets of the organisation, the team and the individual. Translated into a multidisciplinary training programme it will encompass a clear understanding of the 'vision' and goals of the PCG and provide the means for developing all employees so that they are used to their full potential.

Employee relations

All too often 'employee relations' is seen as the arrangements for consultation between management and trade unions or employee representatives. It goes beyond this, however, and should be seen in the wider context of the overall relationship between the employer and employee and the need to have agreed procedures for dealing with different aspects of the relationship at different stages of the individual's employment. In developing its profile as a fair and desirable employer, the PCG, with the aim of ensuring the highest possible standards of employment practice, will need to develop personnel policies and procedures that are consistent with its needs as an organisation and the requirements of employment law. They will, however, also need to be consistently owned and applied with equity by all employers across the PCG. By following agreed policies, managers should know that they are operating with authority and within the law, making decisions consistent with those made by other managers and appropriate to the organisation's fundamental principles. This will be particularly important as PCGs move towards trust status and become the employer of staff previously employed by other organisations with different approaches to employment issues. It is worth noting that where employers have lost cases at an industrial tribunal it has usually been because they have failed either to have personnel procedures which comply with employment legislation or to prove that procedures have been applied consistently and equally within their organisation. If the PCGs can set the ground rules early on in their development, the likelihood of problems occurring when they reach trust status will be lessened.

Recruitment and selection

With changing demographic factors and national shortages of staff in many professions, PCGs must be able to compete within the appropriate labour markets and be seen as attractive organisations within which to work. The human resource strategy should therefore seek to tackle recruitment and retention problems where they exist and to develop new approaches to attracting, keeping and motivating staff.

As employers, PCGs will need to offer equality of opportunity and reflect the ethnic and cultural background of the communities within which they operate. A recent Institute for Professional Develement report[3] highlighted that employers who recruit from a range of backgrounds, including ethnic minorities and people with disabilities, will increase the pool of skills on which they can draw and so increase efficiency as well as contributing positively to the local economic infrastructure. The PCG will need to develop fair and equitable recruitment and appointments processes which will be applicable at all levels of the organisation, providing equal opportunities to all applicants irrespective of their race, creed, sex, marital status, age or disability.

Aligned to this will be the need to develop a fair and equitable system of job evaluation and reward. This will ensure that all staff will have pay, conditions of service and personal development opportunities that are consistent with those of their colleagues doing similar work in other parts of the organisation. This will involve the harmonisation of employment packages and staff benefits across the organisation and guarantee a consistent and equitable approach to prospective employees.

PCGs will also need policies and procedures that outline how as an organisation it will deal with such issues as:

* discipline and grievance
* sickness and absence
* retirement
* staff representation
* equal opportunities
* maternity/paternity leave.

Staff health and welfare

It is now recognised that although its main business is health, the NHS has not always cared properly for the health, safety and well being of its own staff. In recognition of this fact *Our Healthier Nation*[4] and *Working Together*[2] highlight the importance of creating 'healthy workplaces'. As with other employers this will involve the PCG in developing a supportive atmosphere within which to work. This does not mean dealing in a reactive way to meeting the requirements of national and European health and safety legislation, but proactively seeking ways to improve the overall health and quality of life of employees. PCGs may wish to consider for example:

* how they will provide appropriate occupational health services and counselling support for staff
* how they will monitor absenteeism, take action to identify its causes and, where possible, improve sickness absence rates
* how they will monitor and record accidents and incidents of violence against staff and ensure that they have strategies in place to deal with them
* how they will ensure that staff are adequately trained in health and safety issues at induction and regularly throughout employment
* other ways that they can assist staff in improving their overall health and quality of life. An example of this might be to include as part of the employment package subsidised membership of sports clubs or other facilities.

Summary

First class health care delivered by first class staff also requires first class employers. Employers who are committed to involving their staff in decisions on the delivery of services, developing their skills, rewarding them fairly, and providing a good safe working environment free from discrimination and harassment. (A Milburn[5])

The organisational development agenda constitutes a vast programme of work and a steep learning curve for PCGs and there is no doubt that they will require practical help and assistance from experienced human resource professionals to meet the challenges involved. The development of a human resource strategy will be a major prerequisite if the necessary changes are to be achieved and it will play a key role in ensuring that the PCG succeeds as an organisation in the long term.

References

1   Secretary of State for Health (1997) *The New NHS: modern, dependable*. Stationery Office, London.

2   Department of Health (1998) *Working together: securing a quality workforce for the NHS*. Stationery Office, London.

3   Institute for Professional Development. Employment relations in the 21st century. A position paper. IPD, London.

4   Department of Health (1998) *Our Healthier Nation*. Stationery Office, London.

5   Milburn A (1998) Foreword to *Working Together: securing a quality workforce for the NHS*. Department of Health, London.

Further reading

ACAS (1996) *Recruitment Policies for the 1990s*. ACAS, London.

Bramham J (1994) *Human Resource Planning*. IPD, London.

People Management (monthly journal) IPD, London.

Personnel Today (fortnightly journal) Reed Business Info, Sutton.

Reilly P (1996) *Human Resource Planning – an introduction*. Institute of Employment Studies, London.

Appendix: Workforce planning data requirements

Classification	Data type	How it can be used
Information to highlight trends	Staff turnover Staff length of service and stability rates Reasons for leaving Leaver destinations Absentee rates Vacant posts and length of vacancy Sources of recruitment	• For comparison purposes with other local employers • To highlight retention/morale/stress problems • To evaluate recruitment campaigns
Current staff and skills	Staff in post and whole-time equivalents Staff by grade Staff against establishment Staff by work location Staff gender Staff ethnic origin Staff with disabilities Staff by skills and qualifications	• To confirm staffing costs • To monitor full-time/part-time ratios • To indicate recruitment problems/use of budgets • To analyse skills availability • To monitor equal opportunities policy
Information to assist future demand forecasting	Staff age profile Skills required Staff numbers/type required against service plans	• To predict retirement levels • To forecast skills shortages • To highlight need to recruit/redeploy staff
External information	Local labour market information National labour market information Professional organisation registers Local ethnic breakdown Journey-to-work information Local employment statistics Local employers – skills required by Out-turn by education providers	• To analyse availability of skills locally and nationally • To monitor equal opportunities • To analyse/confirm local labour market boundary • To assess competition from other employers

CHAPTER THREE

Education and training

Tim Wilson

Why education and training are so important

The introduction of primary care groups (PCGs) into the 'New NHS' is the greatest challenge facing the 'primary care-led' NHS. For those who have long advocated the concept of organisations such as PCGs they are going to have to prove that they really can run the bulk of NHS services and work in ways that they have never done before. They will have a whole new series of tasks to accomplish. These include:

- working with colleagues in a completely new way (e.g. doctors and nurses on PCG boards)
- working with new partners (e.g. local authorities)
- dealing with a new population scale
- considering the health needs of their patients as opposed to the healthcare needs (e.g. for Health Improvement Programmes).

The only way in which PCGs are going to be able to cope with these tasks, let alone excel and innovate, is if they have a broad range of skills and knowledge, many of which will be new. The suggested skills that PCGs will need immediately are discussed below. There are two options for PCGs:

- ensure that members or employees of the PCG have these skills and areas of knowledge and others are employed or co-opted to fill any gaps; or
- members of the PCG will need to acquire new skills and knowledge after the PCG has started to run.

In truth, like all organisations, they will probably cope by using a combination of these two. Many members of the PCG (board or day-to-day workers) will never have been involved in the management of healthcare; they will need particular help, although they will probably bring new skills and knowledge, which should be valued. Furthermore, not only will PCGs need to ensure they have these skills and areas of knowledge, they will also have to ensure that the skills are kept up to date and added to where needed. This will have to be carefully considered as new members or employees succeed others. If this task were not complicated enough, this education and training agenda needs to complement that of the practice and the individual. These may include important clinical areas, which cannot be neglected because of the needs of the PCG.

Like any large and complex organisation education and training will be crucial. If PCGs do not have the necessary skills and areas of knowledge then they will either fail to succeed or fail altogether. Examples of this are well-documented.[1-3]

Background

The introduction of GP fundholding was the first time GPs had been involved in the commissioning process on a large scale. Other models of primary care commissioning were being developed (locality groups, commissioning, etc.). However, all these methods had one thing in common: the education of the people involved was patchy.[4] Although work was done to try and establish the needs of GPs as commissioners[5] rarely was there a well-established programme of education and training for GP commissioners. Some health authorities ran programmes for GPs and managers involved in commissioning. However, where these courses existed they concentrated on the commissioning process (e.g. negotiation skills, contracting). They tended to concentrate on the lead GP and fund manager, with little thought given to extending the courses to other members of the primary healthcare team or to broadening the subjects to include other skills and areas of knowledge (e.g. joint working skills).

With the growing vogue for evidence-based medicine it became clear that purchasers should develop their skills in finding and applying the evidence, particularly since they increasingly had to justify their decisions on the effectiveness of different therapies. As a result, different courses were developed to promote this, most notably the Critical Skills Appraisal Programme (CASP [6]) and Getting Research into Practice (GRiP[7]). Purchasers were encouraged to develop skills which had traditionally been thought of as public health skills. The CASP courses were extended into newer subject areas and finally included everyone in the primary healthcare team, whether or not they were involved in commissioning. The CASP programme continues; it is being extended into GP commissioning pilots to give board members and stakeholders in these organisations a broad understanding of the ways in which evidence can be used. This will be a useful team-building exercise and confidence building for those with little experience of healthcare management. The way in which this benefits them will prove interesting for PCGs and is being evaluated by the CASP team and the PCG Resource Unit in Oxford.

In summary, education and training has been seen as an afterthought in the 'primary care-led NHS'. It is doubtful whether this is a luxury that can be afforded by PCGs.

Establishing the education and training needs of PCGs

Although there are many parallels with earlier organisations (e.g. total purchasing pilots, commissioning pilots), fundamentally we have a totally new structure. In many ways PCGs have more in common with the way in which health authorities work. Indeed, initially, they will be subcommittees of the local health authority, ultimately responsible to the Chief Executive. Therefore the way in which the best of these organisations ensures a co-ordinate programme of education and training should be studied. However, as already stated, PCGs are completely novel, and apart from the fact they are performing new functions it is this very 'newness' which is important. Much of the education and training will initially concentrate on getting some participants up to speed and, further, will be about the creation of the organisation and the corporate feel that is needed to get participants 'on board'.

What follows is based on the work of the PCG Resource Unit in Oxford. A full copy of the work is available on the Internet.[8] Sensing the confusion about what to do with education and training, the unit set out to try and create a consensus on the education and training needs of PCGs.

Method

Identifying a broad group of interested parties (Box 3.1) across the counties of Bedfordshire, Berkshire, Buckinghamshire, Northamptonshire and Oxfordshire, we canvassed them using the Delphi process. This is a multi-staged survey, the nature of which has been well described elsewhere.[9] Using the responses from one round to construct subsequent rounds, it enables many people to be involved in a powerful and inclusive process. After

---

Box 3.1:   Participants in the education and training consensus

Community and practice nurses
Nurse managers
Nurse education
Educational consortia
GPs
Commissioning and fundholding GPs
GP postgraduate education
Health authority staff and managers
Public health
Those with a specialist interest

two rounds a conference was held. This brought together the participants in the Delphi and other invited interested parties and representatives from national bodies. At the conference the results of the Delphi were collected and further analysed, and then a consensus was established on the education and training needs of PCGs and how they may be delivered.

Important training areas

Three keys areas for education and training are needed:

- creating and running the PCG as an organisation
- planning and management
- public health skills.

These areas are discussed in further detail below. The list is not an exhaustive one but merely highlights the priorities thrown up by the Delphi and conference. There may also be other specific skills needed, which will become more apparent as PCGs develop (e.g. accounting and finance skills).

Creating the PCG as a corporation and making it work together as a team

Box 3.2 shows the skills that were identified as being necessary for the setting up and continued running of the PCG. Some practices have tried to develop them and have used them on 'away days'. Many of these skills are common within the world of industry and larger organisations. Therefore, in some instances it may be worth looking outside the health service to develop these skills. However, failure to develop them within, or import them into (e.g. through the use of facilitators), the PCG may make all the difference between the PCG starting successfully and failing in its first year. If the PCG does not

---

Box 3.2: Skill needed to create and run the PCG

Teamworking and team-building
Understanding the role of others
Co-operation and conflict
Communication (internal and external)
Influencing
Operating as a corporation
Understanding the PCG (including its decision-making mechanisms and its organisation)

---

work as an organisation then it will fail altogether. It would be tempting to miss out the development of skills in this area, concentrating on those in the next two groups. Given the enormity of creating this new corporation it should certainly be a high priority. It should be remembered that the perception of some would be that this is an expensive 'brand promotion' exercise. However, this is in itself a reason to develop the right skills.

Planning and management

Box 3.3 shows the skills needed for planning and management within the PCG. Many of these skills are already held within the healthcare system, most notably within health authorities, GP funds and commissioning. However, some are new (e.g. clinical governance) and the specific training and support for those who need those skills will need particular attention. It is likely that those responsible for clinical governance and other novel areas will need to have regular contact from their colleagues in other PCGs and expert groups (e.g. MAAG). Skills, such as clinical governance, are of course made up of many facets (*see* Chapter 7). However, it is the overall vision and understanding of this concept that will be needed, most importantly by the clinical governance lead.

Box 3.3:   Skills needed for PCG planning and management

Strategic planning
Commissioning
Critical/analytical skills
Project management
Quality management
Clinical governance
Public involvement

Public health skills

The skills needed for public health are shown in Box 3.4. The public health role illustrates the way in which PCGs will have to adopt the 'attitude and perspective' held by public health specialists, that is a broader understanding of health as opposed to healthcare and of dealing with the population as a whole. Health needs assessment is, very often, a skill held by community nurses and so should be encouraged within this group as one important way of including them. However, many will have hardly used their needs assessment skills and will need help to 'resurrect' them.

Note: some of the skills listed within the first two groups could also be categorised as public health skills.

Box 3.4:   Skills needed for public health

Public health role/attitude
Health needs assessment

Common themes to the education and training of PCGs

Possible methods of skill delivery

There are a number of important themes for the delivery of education and training to PCGs.

Training should usually be at PCG level

It is suggested that much training should either be in-post (on-the-job) training or specific training sessions held within the PCG. Not only is this likely to be practical but it will probably ensure good attendance. Furthermore, the training is likely to be highly specific to the needs of the individual or organisation. However, in-house training should not be the only form of training (see below), as mixing with other PCGs and learning away from your place of work is often very rewarding. For instance, there are a number of reasons why specialised training may best be done at multi-PCG level:

- to share experiences between PCGs
- to obtain the best standard of training (a more expensive course or trainer may be used)
- only one or two within the PCG may need some of the most specialised skills.

A co-ordinated curriculum of education and training

A curriculum which considers the needs of the individual, the practice and PCG will be difficult to construct, but is essential. The ability to focus on an individual's learning plan (professional development) and fit that into the needs of a primary healthcare team is only just being achieved by some practices. However, this will need to be extended further and include the needs of the PCG. This theme was expanded in the Chief Medical Officer's report on continuing professional development.[10]

Training should be PCG led

There is no doubt that adult learning should be based on the learner-led principle.[11] PCGs are no exception to this. Based on the co-ordinated curriculum outlined above, the training programme will vary with each PCG because of:

* the different skills and areas of knowledge that those within the PCG have
* the different roles and functions PCGs will take on
* the different pace at which PCGs will evolve. Additionally, running their own education and training programme should give PCG participants a feeling of ownership and therefore greater commitment.

An audit of the skills people already possess and the skills the PCG needs to acquire (on an individual and organisational basis)

Clearly, to co-ordinate the programme for education and training it will be important to find out what skills and knowledge the PCG already has within its members. This must be performed early in the development of the PCG. This will not only be cost-effective but more importantly will ensure that members feel valued and are being asked to do appropriate tasks. Further, it will also allow mapping of the skills and knowledge required by the PCG so a co-ordinated educational programme can be devised. A basic framework consisting of a matrix to complete has been published as part of the Phoenix Agenda.[12]

Perception of need will have to be tempered with actual need

Professionals are not always able to judge what their education and training needs are. There will always be a tendency to obtain education in the style they prefer (which may not always be appropriate) and of the content they are interested in (which very often is not the area they are weakest in). They will need help to decide what their needs are and how they should fulfil them. In particular, clinicians will need help to balance their clinical and managerial development.

Some facilitation will be needed

There will certainly be occasions when the PCG will need to bring in an external facilitator. Those who have run 'away days' for their organisation will understand how there are some areas of development and skill acquisition that can be properly accomplished only by using an external resource. They would not carry the 'baggage' of those within the PCG. This will allow more 'blue sky' thinking (a term commonly used in industry to describe the concept of future planning without the limitations of local horizons). Further, the training skills may be available only from an external resource.

The use of external resources, in particular mentors, is recommended

As stated above, there are likely to be training skills that the PCG does not possess. In particular, it might be valuable to use mentors for certain people within the PCG (e.g. for the knowledge officer of the PCG) who can advise and support them in this new role. These could come from many sources but health authorities and community trusts are likely to be commonly used.

Existing resources, in particular those in health authorities and community trusts, should not be ignored. These organisations often hold a great number of training skills, which should not be wasted. Further, this process would encourage links and the spirit of co-operation needed between PCGs and health authorities and community trusts (important for the PCG as it develops, especially if it has aspirations to trust status itself).

Use existing skills

Within PCGs there will be existing skills for training and education. To find these skills an audit of training and educational skills will be needed, either as people are recruited or later. This will not only be economical but will foster the concept of organisation.

Promote multidisciplinary training

The way in which health workers deliver care is based increasingly on teamwork and changing skill mix; this is probably more true within primary care than anywhere else. As a result, far more training is done as a team (e.g. practice educational sessions). PCGs will have different disciplines performing exactly the same function where they meet on the PCG Board. Also, it is likely that different professional groups working for the PCG (e.g. as a work party) will share skill needs. For these reasons alone, multidisciplinary training will be needed.

There is a degree of suspicion between professional groups regarding the way in which PCGs will run. For instance, there is a fear among doctors that nurses will make decisions that will affect practice finances. In turn, nurses are concerned that doctors will dominate the PCG Board. These concerns should disappear with time as different groups get used to working together and develop a degree of trust and understanding. Multidisciplinary training will greatly hasten this process.

Cross-fertilisation and networking

There will be considerable benefit to PCGs from mixing and sharing ideas. Shared training, especially where sharing ideas is important, will facilitate this. This sharing might involve many members of the PCG on a general course. Alternatively, the course could be specialised and so involve persons within the PCG who have a specific role.

PCGs are likely to have common experiences and difficulties. These should be shared to avoid unnecessary duplication or failures.

Finding the skills to promote 'corporation'

The PCG is a new organisation under development. It is larger than the primary healthcare team (PHCT) but still requires the same level of dedication and ownership that the PHCT evokes. Creating a corporate feeling across the PCG will require new skills, perhaps copied from trusts or industry and commerce. Developing a successful corporate feel will go a long way towards the PCG fulfilling its potential. However, it may well be the most difficult skill a PCG will have to acquire. It is often ignored within the NHS or can be done clumsily (e.g. seemingly spending patient money on the design of the trust logo). Corporation should not mean blind adherence to the 'organisational line' as this is likely to provoke the opposite response from the individuals within it. GPs in particular are a group that dislikes being told what to do. The phrase 'herding cats' has been rather unkindly, but accurately, used. Corporation does mean working towards a common aim and understanding why certain decisions are made. It means supporting the PCG, even when difficult decisions are made. Much of this will be achieved if the individual PCG stakeholders understand the purpose of the PCG and are told clearly why different decisions are being made (i.e. good communication).

The relationship of the Chair and Chief Executive is likely to be crucial. Will the Chief Executive operate in the same way as a clinical manager does in a trust, where the medical director is the lead? Or will he or she operate as the overall leader of the PCG, in the same way the Chief Executive of a trust or health authority works? This is likely to be crucial but will clearly need an entirely different set of skills and knowledge.

Specialist skills

Many of the skills listed above are about how a team or organisation will work effectively. However, there will be some specific skills required (e.g. financial and accounting). These could be identified when the functions of a PCG are known more precisely.

Motivation and attitude

In this chapter the emphasis has been on skills and knowledge. However, it is likely that the attitude and motivation of the participants within a PCG will be more important. Many management experts consider that attitude and motivation have an 80% factor in

---

Box 3.5: Exercise

List the ten attributes you would like to see in someone taking over your job. It is likely that many of these will be attitude-based and only a few to do with skills and knowledge

success and skills only 20%. They cite the effect of motivation on top sports people. And certainly, if considering the factors needed when looking for a top executive, most of them will be attitude (e.g. energy, ambition, etc.) as opposed to their skills.

However, it is estimated that even the best organisations spend only 20% of their time in motivation training and 80% in skills training. It is true that the former is probably more difficult. However, many business experts would recommend altering the emphasis somewhat. PCGs should consider this and not be embarrassed to do so.

The need for an education and training officer within the PCG

Education and training within PCGs needs to be high on the agenda. It also 'needs to be done'. It would be easy to see how it could be the responsibility of no one specific person within the PCG (collusion of anonymity). This is especially true when it might be seen as the responsibility of a number of key persons (e.g. the clinical lead, Chair of the Board, Chief Officer, human resources officer or clinical 'governor'). Although there should perhaps be a committee which brings together interested parties, there will need to be one person who actually makes sure that education and training happens. This person could perform other tasks within the PCG (i.e. they could be the Chief Officer if time permitted). He or she will need to have an interest in education and training and preferably some experience in devising a curriculum and assessing educational needs, and should certainly have access to and report to (if not be a member of) the PCG Board. This is in part because education and training is so important and will need a high priority and funding.

The co-ordination of individual, PHCT and PCG education and training needs will require considerable ability and negotiation skills. Further, bringing together professions in multidisciplinary courses may, initially, be difficult. Like PCG members themselves, education and training officers are likely to have experiences and problems in common with their counterparts in other PCGs. Therefore a grouping of the education and training officers from PCGs would be valuable. It would also be helpful if these groups could have local experts in education and training (e.g. local GP tutors, community trust tutors) who could support, advise and facilitate education and training within PCGs. These 'experts' will need to establish their relationship with the PCG and what each different person does.

The funding of PCG education is unclear, coming as it does from the PCG management allowance, non-medical education and training (NMET), post-graduate medical education (PGME), post-graduate education allowance (PGEA) and development money within health and regional health authorities. This confusing mix will need co-ordination and so it would be useful to have representatives from these organisations attending the education and training officer group meetings.

Conclusions

- Consortia and medical education departments need to co-ordinate action for funding. The funding for education and training in PCGs will come from a number of sources. Because much of the training will be multidisciplinary, the organisations which hold the money for education will need to come together. Otherwise PCGs will find they cannot fund education and training because of bureaucratic problems.
- Education and training needs to be high on the priority list for PCG development at PCG, health authority, regional and national level. Although PCGs should have education and training high on their list of priorities, without support from above they will find it difficult. In particular, the education and training programme within a PCG would be a good marker for performance management.
- The education and training programme should be a 'bottom-up' process led and defined by PCGs themselves, but co-ordination will be needed at all levels (local, regional and national).
- Miss this opportunity to properly equip PCGs with the correct skills and knowledge and at best they will fail to fulfil their potential, at worst they will fail altogether.[2]

References

1 Audit Commission (1996) *What the Doctor Ordered – a study of GP fund holders in England and Wales*. HMSO, London.

2 Wakefield Simulation Exercise (1997) *GPower: the impact of locality commissioning*. Office for Public Management, London.

3 Mays N et al. (1998) *National Evolution of Total Purchasing Pilots*. King's Fund, London.

4 Jones J, Wright J Report of national survey of training for clinicians in commissioning. Personal communication.

5 Harrison D, Wright J (1996) *Developing the GP Commissioning Role*. A report from a workshop held across Berkshire, Buckinghamshire, Northamptonshire and Oxfordshire for the Four Counties Public Health Network.

6 CASP website for a good overview of their project *http://www.ihs.ox.ac.uk/casp*

7 Weston S (1994) *Getting Research into Practice and Purchasing (GRiPP) – a four counties approach*. Resource pack. NHS Executive Anglia and Oxford Region.

8 *http://strauss.ihs.ox.ac.uk/pcgru*

9 Linstone H, Turoff M (1975) *The Delphi Method – techniques and applications*. Addison Wesley, Massachusetts.

10   Department of Health (1998) *A Review of Continuing Professional Development in Practice.* A report by the Chief Medical Officer. DoH, London.

11   Havelock et al. (1995) *Professional Education in General Practice.* Oxford General Practice Series, Oxford University Press, Oxford.

12   NHS Executive (1998) *Phoenix Agenda; a matrix for training needs in PCGs.* NHSE, London.

CHAPTER FOUR

PCGs and commissioning: making the difference

Andrea Young and Mary Wicks

The commissioning role for primary care groups (PCGs) is likely to be shaped by the various models and approaches which have developed over the last ten years, from GP fundholding to total purchasing, locality commissioning and GP commissioning pilots. However, it is a little less clear how things might look ten years from now. In part this is due to political uncertainties, but in the main it is because we are working with an entirely new policy agenda. This new agenda is perhaps more revolutionary than at first appears, especially when put alongside other planned changes in public sector services. However, it is recognised that changes will come about over time, rather than overnight and this is to be welcomed.[1] It means we can learn from our experiences as we move forward; we can invest time in the things that make sustained change, such as developing good working relationships, and it provides the flexibility for organisations and individuals to determine a pace which, while challenging, should not drive people away.

What does this new policy agenda mean for commissioning? For a start it is characterised by collaboration and inclusivity, it is shaped by local needs and based on patients' experiences of health (and social) care, it is explicit about outcomes and is focused on improving quality. What this actually means in practice and how it differs or builds on the previous models will be addressed in this chapter. We will also consider how things could develop in the future and what experiences or learning can be drawn upon.

The White Paper *The New NHS: modern, dependable*[2] sets out a direction of travel for PCG development, including the commissioning function, but essentially sees all PCGs being involved in some way in the commissioning of services for their local population.

Throughout the country there have been a number of different models of commissioning by primary care, including fundholding, total purchasing, GP commissioning pilots, multifunds and locality commissioning projects. By and large GPs have been involved in the business of commissioning through one route or another, so that there is a wealth of valuable experience to build upon. PCGs need to try and retain and sustain the interest of fundholders and commissioning GPs with their teams in developing high-quality services.

Commissioning is essentially a mechanism for defining and shaping the delivery of services. It was introduced into the NHS following the changes brought about by the 1990 NHS and Community Care Act which separated purchasing of healthcare services from provision. It provides a way of focusing service provision on the needs and priorities of the local population. It is argued that much attention was devoted to establishing trusts while the purchasing function was left relatively underdeveloped. Whatever the truth, it is clear that effective commissioning takes time and commitment; it can be difficult but it can also be very powerful in bringing about change.

Commissioning requires a range of skills and it is unlikely that any one person could carry around all this expertise, rather PCGs should be able to bring together a team of people with the relevant skills, at the right time. These skills can be found equally within and outside the PCG. Commissioning should precede or underpin contracts or service and financial frameworks, which set out the financial commitments agreed by all parties. In the past, purchasers directed considerable energies into the contracting process, aiming to negotiate the best deal possible. Fundholders in particular sought marginal gains in getting more activity from providers and indeed were often successful in getting more patients treated. Trusts would try and lower their prices for fundholders to attract business, but needed to shift the real cost on to others or bear the consequences themselves. What emerges is a system characterised by financial and clinical instability, inequity for patients and a focus on money rather than outcomes. While many fundholders were concerned to look at the quality of the services being provided, the consequences for trusts often meant operating different systems for different patients.

The White Paper acknowledges what has been achieved so far, but tries to take us in a new direction. Efficiency and value for money will not go away. But there is a much stronger emphasis on the quality aspects of the service, on developing stability (but not complacency), on working together rather than in competition and in developing solutions in partnership, on providing equitable services within locally agreed strategies. There is devolution of decision making to the local level while retaining a strong central direction of national priorities and clear targets for local health services.

Efficiency will be driven through a number of routes, including national benchmarking of health service prices and, more publicly, through management of waiting times. PCGs will not be able to shy away from this responsibility for too long, but there are opportunities to be gained in looking at the way elective services are accessed and utilised, which PCGs are perfectly poised to tackle. The alignment of clinical and financial responsibility (introduced through GP fundholding and now rolled out on a larger scale) increased emphasis on clinical staff of all disciplines working together and provides a good basis for integrating care across sectors and providers. Recent commissioning guidance from the Department of Health has helped this along further with the drive to develop long-term service agreements managing programmes of care across a number of providers and professionals.[3] The quality markers which fundholders negotiated in their contracts provide an excellent basis to work from and in some cases have underpinned this year's countywide service frameworks.

Expectations of PCGs are high, not withstanding the primary care development side. The responsibility being put at GPs' feet is enormous and many find it overwhelmingly daunting now. But the incentives and levers are in the right place if we can manage to operate them properly and at the right time. Financial control has been given to GPs in recognition of the importance of their relationship to patients and in their role as gatekeeper to other healthcare resources. Unified budgets are often perceived as a threat to primary care but they provide a unique opportunity to reshape services, as costs can be shifted accordingly with the patient flows. The contribution of community nurses on the PCG Board will be invaluable when developing and implementing new community-based services, as well as providing another valuable perspective on patients' needs and community priorities. The lay member also brings the voice of the user and over time this can be developed into a more proactive and structured dialogue. The involvement of social services at board level is extremely important in considering community needs and new service developments.

So far, so good. But what does all this really mean in practice for PCGs operating at the different levels? At level 1, PCGs are to advise the health authority on their commissioning priorities and could work together with other PCGs on a collaborative commissioning project, although they would not be in a position to commit resources. PCGs coming in at this level should take the opportunity to develop an understanding of their local priorities, their budgetary position and where they need to focus their efforts. They will need to ensure they have developed their organisational and managerial capacity to the extent that they are able to make decisions about resources which affect all practices and they should work alongside other PCGs in a co-commissioning role where possible to develop skills and knowledge. Importantly, the role of the health authority will be to ensure that all PCGs are operating within the framework of the Health Improvement Programme (HImP) and that major inequities in service provision are not arising as PCGs develop at different rates. The health authority will also need to closely monitor PCGs' expenditure on prescribing and primary care services (general medical services) at level 1 to ensure financial problems do not arise which cannot then be balanced out through reducing the secondary care budget, and vice versa. Cash reserves and a system for managing risk will need to be applied across all PCGs.

At level 2, PCGs take on responsibility for managing a budget for secondary care services. It is envisaged that over time the whole budget is devolved to PCGs and the recent guidance from the Department of Health[4] set minimum limits for the proportion of the budget to be managed in the next two years. It is likely that the level has been set low in year one to act as a greater incentive to PCGs to move to level 2 immediately, although they will be expected to increase the proportion of the budget over time, and potentially within the financial year. This may create difficulties for the health authority in trying to hold together the whole system.

How might it work in practice? PCGs will need to identify their local priorities at an early stage and then consider the extent to which work on these will also help meet national priorities. Overlap or congruence between the two means less work in the long run and may put the PCG in a better position to accrue additional resources should new money become available nationally. In this first year the government has awarded extra modernisation funding for PCGs through health authorities, if they are able to meet agreed targets or milestones in any of their three functions: improving health, commissioning services, developing primary and community care. This form of incentivisation is expected to be replicated within the PCG to stimulate widespread ownership of and engagement with the PCGs' corporate priorities. For the PCG, incentives will provide an opportunity to demonstrate its ability to make a difference to primary care.

The experience of many total purchasing pilots (TPPs) is that it is harder to achieve change in secondary care, except where it begins to overlap with primary care.[5] For example, TPPs may have been successful in bringing about reductions in length of stay in acute hospitals via discharge co-ordinators or in developing practice-based services such as physiotherapy or podiatry. Choosing an area which is of interest to primary care practitioners is more likely to produce success,[6] and something which makes a difference to the work of the primary care team will in turn generate support for the PCG. Other examples might include near patient testing, a system for booking admissions, specialist community nurses working with practices, enhanced community services to care for older people at home and so on. How do PCGs make a start on these? What are the elements of effective commissioning? The boxes below set out some of the key steps which ought to be considered. But PCGs will need to be pragmatic and take into account the resources available to do the job, the size or scale, and the complexity. PCGs should not shy away from the difficult, but do need to recognise that there would be merits in working collaboratively on large-scale service changes or with seemingly intransigent problems, as well as sharing intentions with the health authority at an early stage to gauge the level of support should the going get really tough. In future years, PCGs' priorities will be rolled up in the HImP, so there should be no surprises or expectations which could be difficult for all parties to deliver.

Many health authorities have also taken a pragmatic view of commissioning, such that areas of major change or those which have been difficult are likely to have been more robustly followed through than those which everyone can sign up to relatively quickly and one is not having to make the case for change at every meeting. The steps in Box 4.1 are a guide to the kind of questions and issues which need to be addressed.

It is clear that different skills and people need to be involved at this stage. Public health expertise can be drawn upon for health needs assessments and for looking at the evidence of best practice and of associated health outcomes. Good information systems and analysts will be required. It is important to build in time to reflect on what emerges from the information at this stage. It may be that the problem is larger than anticipated or that the pattern of service required is not clear cut. However, solutions to the way

---

Box 4.1:   Step 1. Taking stock

Health needs assessment including:
- size of population affected
- population characteristics, e.g. age, sex, ethnicity
- extent to which population is already in contact with services
- health outcomes associated with condition; morbidity and mortality

Review existing services including:
- map existing healthcare provision across spectrum (primary and secondary)
- utilisation rates
- costs
- assessment of quality, user perspectives and hard outcomes
- benchmarking against other providers or alternatives for cost and quality

Other relevant information including:
- what is known about best practice (evidence-based approach)
- how could the service be provided differently?
- what is the scope for change – implications on workforce and for education and training?
- how much will it cost/what are the available resources – can they be deployed differently?

---

forward at this stage can often be more easily found in discussion with others. The involvement of specialists or clinicians at an early stage is important, to test out ideas and different approaches and to get some ownership. This should be considered integral to Step 1.

It is evident that this is a time-consuming and resource-intensive exercise. The key is in matching the scale and complexity of the change or new service being considered with the commissioning work required to implement it. Simple, straightforward changes, such as agreeing different pathological reporting arrangements, will not need the rigour of this approach, nor should simple changes within primary care. In providing a

---

Box 4.2:   Step 2. Reassessing priorities

If there are resource issues it is important to properly identify them before going any further and to ensure the PCG or budget-holding authority is in support. What are the implications for other services, is disinvestment required, or does the service development now depend upon getting additional resources from elsewhere or in the year ahead? Are there economies of scale by getting others involved?

Box 4.3: Step 3. Developing a service specification

Define the service required in terms of:
- describing the nature of the service to be provided
- access, protocols or thresholds
- identifying who is responsible for doing what
- how and where the service is to be provided
- outcomes/quality measures expected
- monitoring information required and review timetable

---

framework for commissioning it is important to recognise that it is only a guide and should not be interpreted as the only way to achieve things. Very often significant achievements happen as a consequence of opportunity, for example the publication of new research. It is important that the commissioning process does not become an obstacle to small innovations that are able to make a great difference to primary healthcare teams, for example the development of phlebotomy services.

The skill for all organisations is maintaining the balance between a focused programme of work which gives everyone a clear sense of direction and measurable objectives, and retaining the capacity to see what's over the horizon and the wider picture. PCGs need to develop their 'antennae' to bring in new ideas and to find out what is happening elsewhere.

What are the keys to success for PCGs?

- Starting with a project that has a scope for making a difference to people working in primary care and where there is some local interest.
- Ensuring management resources are properly identified and bringing in additional help if required.
- Being clear about responsibilities and timescales and reporting progress back to the Board.
- Ensuring that the skills of the Board are being fully utilised.
- Involving nurses in assessing needs and in the planning of new services.
- Exploring the opportunities of providing services differently with social services, specifically around mental health and services for older people.

There is still enormous potential for maximising resources in these areas to improve the service for the patient or user and for reducing cost and bureaucracy. The Government has signalled its support for greater joint working in these areas.[7]

These are the tools to help PCGs on their way, but it is also worth mentioning some of the obstacles to try and avoid disappointments or failure. There will be national imperatives and PCGs may feel they cannot move forward on local priorities with the weight of the 'must dos'. Collaborative commissioning across PCGs will be helpful in making best use of PCG resources and in ensuring consistency and equity across the patch. National service frameworks will provide a clear, well-researched steer for developing local services and are likely to attract additional money for effective local implementation. Resources will always provide limits to what can be done and therefore PCGs should choose a mix of areas to work on, including projects that can be done at a local level led by the Board, those which will require dedicated managerial and clinical time and those involving other PCGs to pool resources. Health authorities obviously have resources in terms of management and specialist advice/skills which need to be made available to PCGs either in a formalised manner,[6] i.e. through dedicated support to individual PCGs, possibly using service level agreements, or by agreeing programmes of work for the year and identifying relative contributions from the PCG and the health authority. These include functions such as strategic planning, project management, development of service specifications, user involvement, finance and costing, public health and financial information. Within primary care there are skills and experience in teamworking, managing staff and budgets, and of knowing what services really make a difference to patients. Other expertise may also be available locally, such as public health resource units, local universities or through local authorities. PCGs at level 3 or 4 may be able to provide certain functions on behalf of the others. It is important that all PCGs get the best management support that they can afford; irrespective of responsibilities, there are a core set of functions required to make any organisation work.[6]

A picture is starting to emerge of a multifaceted approach to PCG commissioning to which has to be added other areas of commissioning, such as the proposed arrangements for specialised services and joint commissioning with social services. With the abolition of the internal market the White Paper introduced new arrangements for specialised services. Specialised services can be defined as those services which do not, in general, treat a large number of patients, they are often accessed in the first instance by a hospital clinician rather than the GP, they are usually high cost, they are at the cutting edge of new techniques or treatments and are not present in every acute hospital. These are for the rare conditions such as haemophilia, or for specialist treatments such as bone marrow transplants. In the past, health authorities were individually responsible for the commissioning of these services and where this was done collaboratively and systematically with neighbouring health authorities, it tended to be more successful.[8] However, there has been a degree of instability for these services, generated both by health authorities taking unilateral action or by trusts developing new services when local need has not warranted that level of provision.

Regional offices of the NHS Executive now have a co-ordinating role to oversee the commissioning of specialised services with local arrangements consisting of four or five health authorities working together with trusts to review the pattern of services across the patch and to provide a co-ordinated and planned approach to commissioning. This subregional role is also likely to encompass quality checks and may include accreditation process over time, similar to the implementation of Calman cancer recommendations. PCGs will need to be involved in this process, although they will not hold the budget for these services. It may be that PCGs will represent each other in these working groups; however, their input is vital, not least because many specialised services impact on general acute services, in terms of the workforce and patterns of care provided, but also because it is important to be able to see the bigger picture in terms of the service being provided across the healthcare system.

For some time health and local authorities have been developing joint commissioning arrangements for services where there is a big overlap between health and social care. Often the stimulus for this way of working can be through the planning of major service change, for example, reprovision of long-stay hospitals, or when there are major budget cuts planned which make it all the more imperative to avoid clients or patients falling between gaps in services as agencies retrench. Streamlining administrative and managerial systems has economic and service benefits.

There will be a degree of joint commissioning in most areas, ranging from joint planning arrangements to pooled budgets with delegated powers given to one authority. PCGs will need to familiarise themselves with these service areas, which are predominantly in the field of mental health, care of older people and for people with learning disabilities. The White Paper envisages community-based mental health and learning disability services potentially moving into primary care trusts, with the more acute or specialised end remaining centrally managed. There are examples of TPPs having established effective joint working with social services regarding the care of older people, to the extent that there are shared budgets accessed by either agency, possibly working from shared premises, e.g. one-stop shops. This approach is being strongly endorsed by the Government, as reflected in the consultation paper on Partnerships in Action and through the National Priorities Guidance for Health and Social Services 1999/00–2001/2. Without specifying one way forward, a number of different models have been proposed for both commissioning and provision of services to be appropriately developed around local arrangements. The social services board member is pivotal to PCGs taking forward this agenda, with major gains to be made for patients and professionals alike.

The White Paper and subsequent guidance has emphasised the importance of PCGs working collegiately around a number of functions. Elements of secondary care commissioning are particularly appropriate to consider in this respect for several reasons. First, there is the concern about financial risks to PCGs taking on responsibility for commissioning certain services where demand is difficult to predict or manage, where services may be expensive and where the actions of one PCG can significantly affect others. This can result in financial and clinical instability within healthcare providers and inequity among users. The experience of TPPs and GP fundholders has been that their purchasing power or leverage to create change in acute hospital services was often weak.[5] A federation of PCGs similar to GP commissioning forums, or fundholding consortia working together on secondary care commissioning could realign the balance of power. In strategic terms the HImP will set some parameters to the extent and range of service change envisaged, but this should not be an excuse for maintaining the status quo. It is important that PCGs do take risks at times and that they are properly equipped to do so.

PCGs of 100 000 population will have a sizeable budget to manage some of the financial risks associated with secondary care commissioning. But if they are all focused on doing the same things separately they will not make the difference needed at a higher level. Alternative arrangements could include one PCG employing core staff on behalf of the other, more likely at level 3 or 4, or some support contracted in from other agencies. Health authority management resources will transfer over time to PCGs, but this comes with all the attendant responsibilities. While larger PCGs may have greater flexibility in their budgets, their organisational arrangements also become more complicated. PCGs should also fully utilise the wealth of resources within their primary healthcare teams, providing cross cover for practices, backed up with appropriate education and training.

In the first year, PCGs should set themselves a range of objectives which include some easy wins – those developments which may be small-scale, locally generated and primary care-focused. But they should also gain experience in the more complex areas, to gain exposure and the confidence to take on more over time. This will be achieved through effective collaboration with health authorities and in an environment which is supportive and facilitative rather than defensive. Good relationships with health authorities have been cited by many TPPs as an important factor in their success.[5] So what might a future look like with PCGs in the driving seat of commissioning? There are likely to be less PCGs than we have now, with mergers taking place, hopefully in a planned way. At primary care trust level we may begin to see bodies resembling the American model of health maintenance organisations, combining the provision of high-quality primary care, patient education and active promotion of self-care with commissioning of expensive hospital services. These organisations arose in response to frustrations by the insurance companies who were trying to contain costs and expenditure on healthcare, but who did not have the knowledge, expertise, scale of budget or facilities to redirect patients into other, more appropriate and cost-effective forms of healthcare.[9] PCGs have the knowledge, the know how and the unified budget to make this a serious proposition. In England the development of commissioning by PCGs takes us towards a truly primary care-led NHS.

References

1   Parston G, McMahon L (1998) A third way? England – yes; Scotland – maybe. *BMJ.* **316**: 214.

2   Secretary of State for Health (1997) *The New NHS: modern, dependable.* Stationery Office, London.

3   NHS Executive (1998) *Commissioning in the New NHS.* HSC 1998/198. NHSE, London.

4   NHS Executive (1998) *The New NHS Modern and Dependable. Primary Care Groups: delivering the agenda.* HSC1998/228:LAC(98)32. NHSE, London.

5   Mays N, Goodwin N, Killoran A et al. *Total Purchasing. A Step Towards Primary Care Groups. National Evaluation of Total Purchasing Pilot Projects.* King's Fund, London.

6   Killoran A, Griffiths J, Posnett J et al. (1998) *What Can We Learn from the Total Purchasing Pilots about the Management Costs of Primary Care Groups?* A briefing paper for health authorities. King's Fund, London.

7   *Partnerships in Action. New Opportunities for Joint Working between Health and Social Services.* (1998) A discussion document. Stationery Office, London.

8   Audit Commission (1997) *Higher Purchase: commissioning specialist services in the NHS.* Audit Commission, London.

9   Light D (1998) Is NHS purchasing serious? An American perspective. *BMJ.* **316**: 217–20.

CHAPTER FIVE

Communication and involving stakeholders

Elaine Richardson

Effective communication is the key to any relationship. Yet it is an area where all too often little attention is paid until problems become evident. Primary care groups (PCGs) need to invest time and energy in the area of communication as the success of the PCG will depend on the quality of its relationships. Laing and Cotton[1] describe communication as the 'lynchpin of effective operations' in GP fundholding consortia and suggest it was the area that individual practices identified consortia as failing to manage effectively.

In the area of communications, the adage 'failing to plan is planning to fail' is very appropriate. So while it may not seem to be high on the priority list, developing a communications strategy for the PCG should be one of the first tasks of the Chief Officer. The implemented strategy will then support every aspect of the work of the PCG. The aim of this chapter is to outline the issues that need to be considered when developing and then implementing a communications strategy. Health authorities, trusts and regional offices are likely to have communication experts who will be willing to help and they may even have a strategy that can be adapted.

Developing a communications strategy

The strategy will answer four fundamental questions:

- Why does the PCG need to communicate?
- What does the PCG need to communicate?
- Who needs to be involved in PCG communication?
- How will the PCG communicate?

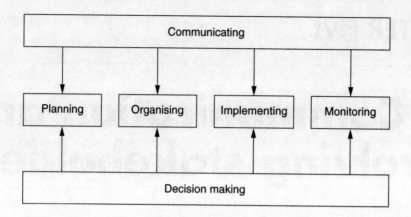

Figure 5.1: The management context. Taken from Murdock and Scutt.[2]

Why does the PCG need to communicate?

That the individuals and organisations that make up a PCG will need to communicate with each other in order to carry out the work of the PCG almost goes without saying, but such internal communication is a vital part of the communications strategy. Murdock and Scutt[2] describe communication as 'a critical component of almost every management skill', which they demonstrate through Figure 5.1.

HSC 1998/139 reinforces the need for communication in the management of PCGs when it states that boards 'must seek to include all those who have a legitimate interest and who wish to be directly involved in the policy and decision making process'[3] and that structures should 'promote the involvement of a wider range of staff where experience and expertise is vital to the development of high quality services'.[4]

However, it is not only internal communication that needs to be considered. External communication is also going to be important for PCGs as they are expected to work in partnership with other NHS organisations and local authorities and be responsive to their stakeholders, including the public.

Some organisations choose to treat internal and external communication differently, some even have separate strategies. However, PCGs would do well to treat them the same and integrate them both throughout the strategy.

The answer to the question of 'Why?' can be summarised as 'to gain involvement' and this becomes the aim of the communications strategy. The objectives are then likely to include:

- to develop trust and confidence among all stakeholders
- to impart information in a way that enables the PCG to function effectively
- to gain information from stakeholders in order to achieve synergy
- to influence stakeholders to bring about change.

These objectives then start to inform the next question when what it is that needs to be communicated is considered.

What does the PCG need to communicate?

The 'What?' aspect of the strategy is not about the specifics that will need to be communicated, as these will vary, but about the categories the specifics will fall into. Categories such as:

- **Organisational**: relating to the PCG as an organisation. Including issues such as: what it is; who is involved; its structure; its aim.
- **Managerial**: relating to how the PCG will achieve its aim. Including issues such as: roles and responsibilities; employment information; policies; decisions that have been made.
- **Team**: relating to how individuals in the PCG get the work done. Including issues such as: working on a project; research information; problem solving; reaching a decision.
- **Social**: relating to the fact that when people work together social interaction occurs. Including issues such as personal information.

Recognising that there are different categories helps prevent both absence of communication and communication overload as each can be related to the various people involved in communication and links made as to who will be involved at each level. It also allows different means of communication to be employed. An issue for PCGs will be confidentiality, as some information will be inappropriate to share. This also needs to be considered when exploring who is involved in communication.

Who needs to be involved in communication?

Communication is a two-way process even though one party will usually instigate it. Successful PCGs will develop communication systems that enable any stakeholder to instigate and be involved in communication. Considering who needs to be involved in communication rather than who the PCG will communicate with fosters that approach. There are many different players in the game of communication as summarised in Figure 5.2, all of which will have variable needs.

Every one of the players in Figure 5.2 has a responsibility for communication, but just leaving it up to each individual is rarely effective and can lead to misinformation. Because of the wide range of audiences, having someone with overall responsibility for co-ordinating communication could be very useful. This does not mean that everyone else can abdicate his or her own responsibility but it helps to ensure a more co-ordinated

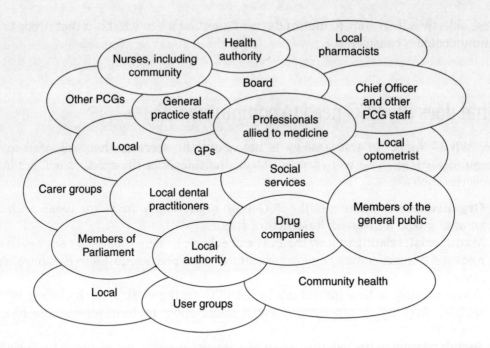

Figure 5.2:   People involved in PCG communication.

approach, especially in the early days. Having a centralised communications structure
was shown to be an effective way for groups to achieve simple tasks by Baron and Greenboys.[5] They used Shaw's centralised structure of a wheel and decentralised structure of
a comcon (Fig 5.3) and compared the level of task performance.

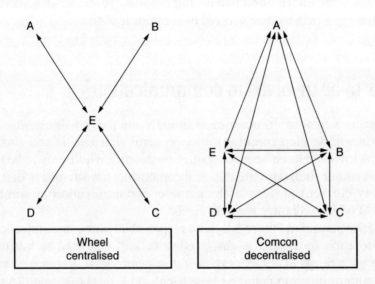

Figure 5.3:   Shaw's communication networks. Taken from Huczynski and Buchanan.[5]

In simple tasks the individual at the centre of the wheel (E) has all the information they need to perform effectively, whereas in the comcon it is very hard for any one person to have all the information. Effectiveness is reversed when the task is a complex one, as in the wheel the central person becomes overloaded but in the comcon everyone shares the burden and works together to achieve a successful outcome.

The communications co-ordinator will therefore be most effectively used to advise on the most appropriate method of communication and support those methods that involve considerable organisation, e.g. meetings, media contact or newsletters. A named contact will also be useful as it is easier to contact a specific person rather than having to guess where to start. However, he or she should not be expected to manage all communication.

It is easy to forget that individuals within PCGs need to communicate with themselves as well as with others. This may seem to be a strange thing to include in a communications strategy, but unless people first think through issues for themselves they may be unclear about what they wish to communicate. Failing to invest in personal thinking time generally leads to a waste of team time. This situation is seen at many meetings when people have not thought about the issues on the agenda or read the papers, so discussion is difficult and the group are finally asked to come back to it again or comment separately at a later date. Giving credibility to thinking time through setting standards for the methods of communication may help prevent it getting squeezed out when time becomes pressured.

How will the PCG communicate?

Like the 'What?' question this is not about specifics but more about principles. One way of identifying the principles for effective communication is to look at how it can fail.

Murdock and Scutt highlight the barriers to effective communication that have been identified by the Open University[6] and these point to ten principles (Table 5.1). If an overriding principle of 'Prepare and plan properly' is adopted, the barriers can be overcome. The ten principles in Table 5.1 then become the process by which the proper preparation and planning takes place.

A good PCG communication strategy will follow the keep it short and simple (KISS) principle and should last for five or more years. Its aim and objectives are unlikely to change as long as there is an NHS and neither are the What, Who and How, as they are general rather than specific. The strategy really describes the process that all communicators should go through to ensure effective communication.

The detail lies not in the strategy but in the implementation plan, which may well change, as new technologies become available and the environment changes.

Implementing the strategy

This section contains a mixture of suggestions as to how the strategy can be implemented and further detail on the principles.

Table 5.1:   Barriers to and principles of effective communication

Barrier		Principle
Uncertainty of message	1	Be clear about what you wish to communicate
Unstated assumptions Incompatible viewpoints	2	Seek first to understand then to be understood
Cumulative distortion	3	Use direct communication wherever possible
Interference	4	Seek to get feedback
	5	Make communication timely
Deception	6	Be open and honest
Limited capacity of audience	7	Keep it short and simple (KISS)
	8	Involve the left and right brain
Faulty presentation	9	Use competent and capable communicators
Lack of channels	10	Use all the opportunities for communication as appropriate

When planning individual communications the first thing to do is think through what you wish to communicate; however, one of the most useful things a PCG can start doing straight away is to concentrate on the 'Who' and compile a database of contacts. The format for the database should be one that can be easily used for as many communication methods as possible, e.g. a computer file that can be easily accessed, updated, manipulated, used in mail merges and, if necessary, printed. Whatever format is used, care must be taken to ensure that the information on it is appropriate and that the Data Protection Act is not violated. There must be someone responsible for initially checking and then maintaining its accuracy if it is to be used effectively. Inaccurate databases immediately violate the principle of being clear about what you wish to communicate as they communicate lack of attention to detail, lack of interest in the individual and possible incompetence, not something most PCGs would like to be communicating.

Be clear about what you wish to communicate

The above example highlights the fact that the message we communicate is made up of many different aspects. Albert Mehrabain's research on how a message is communicated in face-to-face situations attributes 7% to the words, 38% to voice tone and 55% to body language[7] and even when using the written word the visual presentation will communicate a great deal. So concentrating on the words used to communicate is important but not to the exclusion of the other aspects of the message.

One area where visual presentation is usually accepted as an important channel of communication is that of corporate identity. While PCGs will need to behave as corporate bodies, they are still subcommittees of the health authority so will need to reflect the corporate identity of the health authority. Names, house styles and logos can help communicate a corporate identity but are complex areas, fraught with dangers and expensive pitfalls. PCGs would be wise to wait and work with their health authorities to plan how they can promote their corporate identity in a cost-effective way.

There will be many other messages that PCGs will have to communicate, both strategic and operational. In all situations, investing time in thinking through the message will be vital, as communicating the wrong message is at best costly and at worst destructive.

Seek first to understand, then to be understood

This principle is described by Stephen Covey as the single most important principle in effective interpersonal communication.[8] He suggests that only when you understand an audience can you present your own ideas in a way that relates to them. He cites the advantages as 'greater accuracy and greater integrity in your presentation' with people knowing that 'you're presenting the ideas which you genuinely believe, taking all known facts and perceptions into consideration, that will benefit everyone'. These advantages are important for PCGs as it is going to be impossible to please everyone and hard decisions are going to have to be made. This principle will need to operate in the day-to-day functioning of the PCG if stakeholder involvement is to be secured.

Some people see discussion as the mechanism for giving people the chance to be heard but Bohm and Covey warn of its dangers. Bohm[9] likens discussion to a table tennis game with the subject being analysed and dissected from the points of view of those taking part and the fundamental purpose being to get one's own views accepted by the group. Covey[10] confirms this by suggesting that when listening, most people are not listening in order to understand but in order to reply, so they filter things through their own paradigms whilst preparing to speak. Peter Senge[9] sees dialogue as the process by which the principle can be achieved, where people suspend their assumptions while communicating them freely so the full depth of people's experience and thoughts are surfaced. This, he believes, leads to the free flow of meaning between people and enables genuine 'thinking together' so that understanding goes beyond any one individual, that is synergy occurs.

Developing dialogue is not an easy option but one worth working at because, as Figure 5.4 summarises, it links two of the other important factors required for successful PCGs.

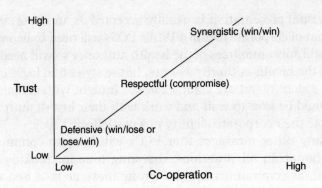

Figure 5.4: Developing dialogue: levels of communication. Reprinted with permission from Covey S (1994).[11]

Use direct communication whenever possible

The principle of using direct communication wherever possible is based on the fact that the overall aim of communication for PCGs is to achieve involvement, and evidence shows that shared visions tend to develop through personal contact. Direct written communication does have its place but it does not guarantee the co-operative communication that tends to develop through face-to-face relationships. HSC 1998/139[12] sees meetings as being an important channel of communication and suggests that PCGs use open meetings as a way of enabling people to see how decisions are made. Unfortunately many people feel that meetings are a waste of time, especially when transport time is included, but they do have an important role which cannot be substituted by other forms of communication. It will therefore be important for PCGs to develop the skills and discipline needed to hold effective meetings.

Cascade systems will be necessary in PCGs as it will be impossible to communicate directly with everyone on everything. They can work well, provided people remember that the person cascading the message will have interpreted the original according to their own beliefs, values and experiences. This takes us back to the first principle and the need to reflect on what the message is. The person cascading the message must check out the bias they are giving the message. This is particularly important for those individuals acting in a representative role, e.g. board members. One way of helping overcome bias is to have people jointly cascading so they can work together to reduce the bias.

Seek to get feedback

This principle helps the communicator establish the effect the personal filters of the audience have had and whether the message has been understood as he or she intended.

It closes the loop of communication. One way of getting feedback is for the instigator of the message to ask questions. In meetings, an important role of the chair is to summarise discussions and decisions and this can highlight any different interpretations of what was said. With written communication it is more difficult to get feedback, especially immediately. This is why written communication is best used to communicate straight-forward and simple messages that are unlikely to be easily misinterpreted.

Make communication timely

The timing of communication involves two issues: timeliness, that is ensuring messages are communicated at the time they need to be, and appropriateness, that is ensuring they are communicated when the appropriate people are there. Both are likely to present problems for PCGs as PCG work will be to some extent in addition to the day-to-day work of the stakeholders.

Mintzberg[13] suggests that the reason why managers strongly favour verbal media – namely, telephone calls and meetings – is because it helps them gain information that is more timely. Ensuring that messages are communicated at the right time helps prevent miscommunication and conflicting messages but it involves planning. Having regular meetings will ensure that most routine communication can be handled, with the frequency of the meetings depending on their purpose. However, unexpected or urgent communications will be more difficult as it may be problematic to get people together at short notice. Developing a system using electronic mail or faxes will enable more instantaneous communication but will restrict the messages that can be sent. This, however, may well be better than no communication at all.

There is no easy answer to the problem of communicating at an appropriate time. With regular meetings it pays to arrange the first and then agree with all involved a mutually acceptable pattern and keep to it. Even the timing of meetings sends out a message. For example, evening meetings may suggest that the subject is less important than work or that it is so important that social time will be sacrificed. The key is to explore the interpretation those involved have put on the timing, not just to assume they haven't attributed one. When the PCG instigates communication with the general public, it should consider when may be a good time for the public rather than when can the PCG do it. Too often if a public meeting fails to attract the public it is assumed that they are not interested when it may simply be that the timing was not convenient.

Be open and honest

Hilarie Owen, in her book about the Red Arrows[14] highlights how the principle of open and honest communication enables the team to fly the way it does. By having meetings where all the team adopts this principle when talking through issues, a sense of trust is developed. This trust then enables a pilot to manoeuvre his plane without first having to check that another member of the team has moved his. Trust will be very important for PCGs, as without the trust it is unlikely that decisions will be implemented.

To be open with others it is first necessary to be open and honest with ourselves, and this takes confidence. PCGs already have experience of moving forward into the unknown and some have had the confidence to cope when health authorities have admitted they do not know the answers, whereas others have still pushed for an answer. Admitting they don't know all the answers and that PCGs are a learning experience will be important if PCGs are to operate openly and honestly.

Communications that avoid the use of generalisations and sweeping statements tend to promote a greater honesty. For example, a GP who states 'GPs do not believe...' usually closes down a discussion, unless there is another more forceful GP who will challenge, whereas stating 'I do not believe...' invites others to comment.

To be open and honest, individuals must believe their contribution is valued and that there is no danger of ridicule or retaliation. The chair of a meeting must create an atmosphere that encourages such openness and honesty.

Keep it short and simple (KISS)

The NHS is notorious for its use of jargon and most PCGs recognise the need to try to avoid it or at least explain it. The KISS principle reinforces that need and reminds us that people's time and attention spans are limited. In presentations, it is better to keep it short and allow time for questions rather than making such a long presentation that the audience switches off before the end. In meetings, the discipline of setting time frames for discussions can help the chair as it tends to prevent people waffling and straying from the subject. Setting a limit on the length of written communication is another useful discipline as it forces the writer to plan carefully. This not only helps the reader understand the message but also makes it easier to find time to read the document. Four sides of A4 is a reasonable limit to the length for many management papers, as any supporting documentation can be made available if required. When planning written communication, measures such as the Flesch Readability Index may be helpful in checking the readability of the text. Many word processing packages now contain automatic spelling, grammar and readability tests.

It has been said that a picture paints a thousand words so using visuals can be helpful in this principle. However, if they need too much explanation they become redundant so should be avoided.

Involve the left and right brain

The principle of involving the left and right brain helps prevent those you are communicating with from switching off while at the same time developing a more complete message. Empathic listening described by Covey[15] as the type of listening that is necessary for effective communication involves both the left and right brain. To use Covey's words 'You sense, you intuit, you feel'.

Typically the left side of the brain deals with logical issues, such as language, mathematics, reading and sequencing, and the right side with visual images and feelings. Written communication tends to appeal to the left brain, which is why diagrams and pictures are one way of following this principle. However, it is not just actual pictures or diagrams that can be used but also verbal ones such as metaphors. Face-to-face communication lends itself more easily to this principle as it is easier to use visuals. But if the verbal message is purely prose it will only engage the left brain. Anecdotes, metaphors and rhymes are all verbals that appeal to the right brain.

The above still tend to focus on sight and hearing and if a way were found to exploit the other three senses the potential for impact would be even greater. Whilst this idea may seem too far-fetched for PCGs, it is important to ensure that the remaining three senses do not have a destructive impact on PCG communication. For example the message may be completely lost if communicated to an audience sitting on hard plastic chairs in a cold room next to the kitchen around lunchtime.

Advertising exploits the left/right brain principle and may provide some useful ideas for PCGs when considering how to achieve this principle.

Use competent and capable communicators

Bert Decker suggests 'The key ingredient to effective communication is credibility'.[16] This links to the second principle of 'seek first to understand' and its importance for PCGs. Unfortunately getting this principle wrong not only violates the second, it is also likely to violate the first principle. Thankfully communication skills can be learnt, the problem is getting people to recognise they need to learn them. Listening is a classic example. The listening skills of most people are only 25% effective even though 40% of communication activities involve listening. Yet listening is the least taught communication skill with between zero and one/two years being devoted to formal training.[17] While a broad-brush approach to training and development is not usually recommended, it may be the best way for PCGs to tackle this area. The process of communicating the communications strategy could itself be used to develop the level of communications skills within the PCG.

Board members must lead by example ensuring that their own communication skills are developed to a high level and that they use them effectively.

Use all the opportunities for communication as appropriate

There are many channels of communication, as Figure 5.5 shows. Unfortunately, very often particular channels are used without really considering why. One of the key issues for PCGs will be to consider first what they need to communicate, then whom they need to communicate with and finally how, to ensure that the most appropriate channel is

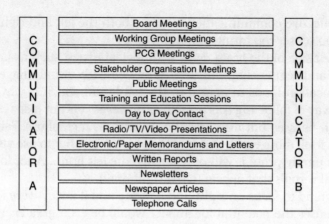

Figure 5.5: Communication channels available to PCGs.

used. For example, to invite the general public to a meeting a PCG needs to communicate details of what the meeting is for as well as when and where it is to all the people covered by the PCG. An advert in the local newspaper, on local radio, in community areas such as shops, the library or bus station, plus possibly house-to-house leaflets will be more effective than word of mouth or putting an advert in practices alone.

Reaping the rewards

Communication is a means to an end not an end in itself. It is a strategic activity. PCGs will need to invest considerable effort and resources into developing effective communications but the return on that investment will be high, as it will create trust, reduce misunderstandings, facilitate job satisfaction, ensure efficiency and success, and involve all of the stakeholders.

References

1   Laing A, Cotton S (1997) Partnerships in purchasing: development of consortium-based purchasing among GP fundholders. *Health Services Management Research.* **10**: 245–54.

2   Murdock A, Scutt C (1995) *Personal Effectiveness.* Butterworth Heinemann, Oxford, p 12.

3   NHS Executive (1998) *Developing Primary Care Groups.* HSC 1998/139. NHSE, London, p 11.

4   NHS Executive (1998) *Developing Primary Care Groups.* HSC 1998/139. NHSE, London, p 16.

5   Baron and Greenboys (1991) In: A Huczynski, D Buchanan *Organisation Behaviour: an introductory text* (2e). Prentice Hall, New York, pp 205–7.

6   Murdock A, Scutt C (1995) *Personal Effectiveness.* Butterworth Heinemann, Oxford, p 24.

7   Mehrabain A (1968) Communication without words. *Psychology Today.* September: 53.

8   Covey S (1994) *The Seven Habits of Highly Effective People.* Simon and Schuster, New York, p 237.

9   Senge PM (1993) *The Fifth Discipline: the art and practice of the learning organisation.* Century Business, London, pp 240–1.

10 Covey S (1994) *The Seven Habits of Highly Effective People.* Simon and Schuster, New York, p 239.

11 Covey S (1994) *The Seven Habits of Highly Effective People.* Simon and Schuster, New York, p 270.

12 NHS Executive (1998) *Developing Primary Care Groups.* HSC 1998/139. NHSE, London, p 14.

13 Mintzberg H (1975) The manager's job: folklore and fact. In: DS Pugh (ed) *Organizational Theory: selected readings* (1990) Penguin Books, Harmondsworth, p 287.

14 Owen H (1996) *Creating Top Flight Teams.* BCA, London, pp 99–103.

15 Covey S (1994) *The Seven Habits of Highly Effective People.* Simon and Schuster, New York, p 241.

16 Decker B (1993) *How to Communicate Effectively.* Kogan Page, London, p 27.

17 Burley-Allen M (1982) *Listening: the forgotten skill.* John Wiley & Sons Inc, Chichester, p 31.

Further reading

Heylin A (1993) *Putting it Across: the art of communicating, persuading and presenting.* Michael Joseph Ltd, London.

Honey P (1997) *Chairing Meetings: questionnaires for 360° feedback.* Honey Publications.

Mandel S (1992) *Effective Presentation Skills.* Kogan Page, London.

Pedlar M, Burgoyne J, Boydell T (1994) *A Manager's Guide To Self Development* (3e). McGraw-Hill, London.

CHAPTER SIX

Information requirements

Bruce Donn

Introduction

Primary care groups (PCGs) will be extremely information-hungry organisations. It is inconceivable that the kinds of plans and decisions they will need to make won't be based on a solid foundation of relevant information. And they will have high demands for simple and effective communications with a wide range of other organisations.

In the early days of the development of PCGs much will need to be done regarding information, but there are uncertainties about exactly how PCGs will look in a few year's time. This poses something of a dilemma. The golden rule for information systems is to be clear about the business objectives and functions *before* you start planning your systems solutions.

The NHS strategy *Information for Health*[1] defines an ambitious programme of NHS-wide developments which have electronic health records and electronic communications at their heart. There is much that is relevant to the needs of PCGs, but it will take the next 5–10 years to implement. The message for PCGs must be to position themselves to exploit these strategic developments and to shape them to meet their needs as the PCG role evolves, while finding pragmatic solutions for the short term.

This chapter focuses on the needs of PCGs rather than on the operational and clinical needs of primary care, although there are clearly important relationships between the two. It aims to steer a path between pragmatism and future-gazing, by asking:

- Why do PCGs need information?
- What sorts of information are needed, from what sources?
- What things need to borne in mind when using these types of information?
- What are the communications needs of PCGs, and some possible solutions?

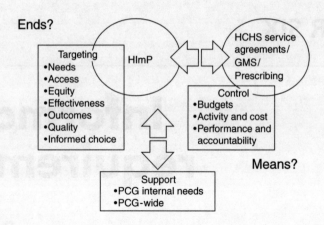

Figure 6.1:   PCG functions.

What will PCGs do?

If we want information and systems to add value to the PCG business, we need to have some fix on the range of functions that information and communications systems may need to support. Chapters 4 and 8 discuss the principal PCG roles of improving health, commissioning secondary care and developing primary care. Figure 6.1 groups the various functions under three broad headings: control, targeting and support.

One of the key messages from the analysis below is that although 'bean-counting' associated with 'control' functions is important, the effort it takes needs to be carefully balanced against the wider information and communications needs. The high trans-action costs associated with data collection and validation for fundholding, for example, will not be tenable for PCGs. Therefore monitoring mechanisms must be developed which are less onerous in terms of effort. The 'ring-fencing' of this 'control' activity will represent a challenge to PCG managers.

Control activities are focused around the balancing of targets for activity and expend-iture across the unified budget – for secondary care, for primary care and for prescribing. The key drivers are financial control and statutory accountability. Monitoring activities in relation to secondary care are familiar to those involved with fundholding and total purchasing projects (TPPs). However, the scope covered by PCGs clearly is much broader. Clinical governance will require PCGs to monitor key aspects of service quality.

PCGs are likely to have an important role in reviewing primary care expenditure pat-terns examining issues such as overheads for management and premises against targets, for example for population screening, immunisation, child health surveillance and other quality measures. Primary care prescribing accounts for a substantial proportion of the unified budget, therefore understanding and influencing the variations in prescribing among practices and against national norms will be of interest.

Targeting is the public health agenda, where local priorities for health-gain feed into and reflect the local Health Improvement Programme (HImP). Key activities will include needs assessment, setting local health gain targets, reviewing service provision options and planning future services. The primary drivers will be the need to ensure positive outcomes from equitable and effective interventions. Many of these issues will be difficult to measure, and the processes will involve many organisations within and outside healthcare.

The possible *support* activities of PCGs are twofold. First, the PCG will need to spend time covering its own administrative needs, e.g. administering meetings and maintaining its internal accounts. Second, as part of its clinical governance remit, the PCG could play an important role in identifying and facilitating best practice within primary care. The PCG also provides an opportunity for practices to share resources, so the facilitation role could include organising training for practice-based staff, facilitating discussion groups, mentoring or co-ordinating arrangements in specialist areas such as IT support, all of which have communications components.

Information requirements

Box 6.1 illustrates the diversity of issues which PCGs may seek to address by posing some hypothetical questions. Every question the PCG seeks to address needs to be underpinned by information. Some of these information points are identified in Box 6.1.

Box 6.1:   Some possible questions

Control
  - What are the reasons for 'overperformance' within our main general medicine service agreement? Is the known increase in respiratory tract infections solely responsible?
Information points: admissions data from trust; examine case mix, using Healthcare Resource Groups;[2] compare with expected patterns from historical data
  - Are high numbers of asthmatic patients being admitted, indicating inappropriate condition management within primary care?
Information points: admissions data from trust; analyse admission rate per practice for asthma main diagnosis; age/sex standardisation; examine distribution of rates (see Figure 6.2)
  - Are some practices prescribing unacceptably high levels of drugs which are not on the agreed local formulary?
Information points: PACT data; table of formulary drugs; analyse % distributions; 'drill down' into data for practices in the top 10%.

Box 6.1: Continued

Targeting
- Has health status or perceptions of health changed within the population of 'Green Acres' estate since the housing improvement programme was implemented?

Information points: Work with local authority; questionnaire survey before and after changes; lifestyle and health status scores such as 'SF-36'[3]
- Are all patients with hypertension given special advice on diet?

Information points: clinical audit within primary care team; practice-held data; systematic data recording; Read codes;[4] analysis tools such as MIQUEST[5]
- Is our PCG's hysterectomy rate higher than for the rest of the country? Is it reducing?

Information points: National admission rates via Office for National Statistics (ONS); local data pooled across PCGs; hospital admission rates by main procedure; age standardised; time series
- Is our population experiencing higher levels of mortality from heart disease than would be expected from the county population as a whole?

Information points: local standardised mortality ratios from ONS data files; analyse local data by postcode; approximate mapping of postcodes to PCG boundaries; several years' data to counteract small numbers
- Are female residents of our population between the ages of 30 and 65 satisfied with the range and quality of breast screening and breast care services provided for them?

Information points: no routine data; questionnaire survey; practice registers; information from voluntary groups; complaints statistics; need statistically valid sample sizes (see Figure 6.3)

Support
- Are our local GPs aware of latest evidence on best practice for management of asthma?

Information points: NHSnet access to National Electronic Library for Health/National Institute for Clinical Effectiveness; compare with local database of guidelines and protocols; disseminate advice to all practices

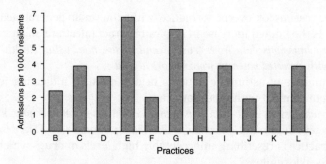

Figure 6.2: Variation in hospital admissions between practices within a PCG for childhood asthma, a condition which should be predominantly dealt with by primary care (data are for illustrative purposes only).

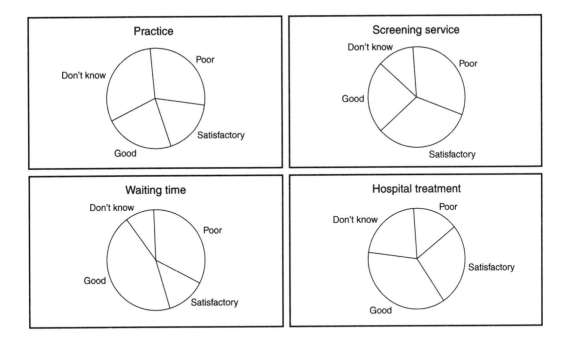

Figure 6.3: Women's views about the quality of four different aspects of services to support breast cancer screening and care (data are for illustrative purposes only).

Health intelligence

The examples above illustrate the tremendous spread of information needed to support the diverse PCG roles. Much of the information needed is not 'transactional' (i.e. used to support a specific process such as paying an invoice, as in fundholding) but can be classed as health 'intelligence', used to make decisions and to investigate particular problems. Areas of investigation will change over time.

Figure 6.4 illustrates that intelligence information is anything it needs to be! It may be derived from routine sources or collected from specially designed surveys and sampling. It may be largely numerical, or it could be largely textually based, such as literature reviews on the effectiveness of certain treatments. Some information will need to be held locally, much will be accessed from others, including library services, the Internet and local intranets.

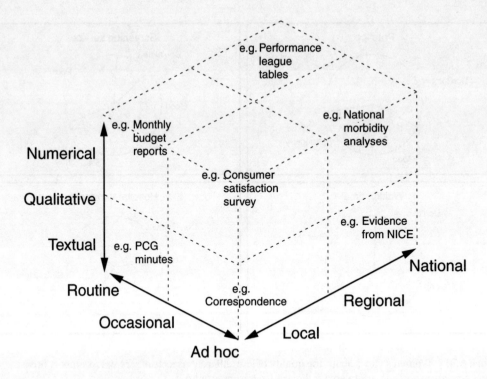

Figure 6.4: Diversity of health intelligence information.

Performance review

The New NHS defines the areas within which performance will be assessed. Measures for these will be codified in a new national framework for assessing performance.[6] PCGs may need to monitor their performance in various areas and report to their health authority (*see* Table 6.1).

Clinical governance

A First Class Service[7] describes the need for all parts of the NHS to follow 'best clinical practice'. There are two important associated information issues for PCGs:

• The need to know where each service stands in relation to national norms. This implies a much greater use of comparative data, e.g. to examine variation in

Table 6.1:   Monitoring performance

Performance area	Possible examples of monitoring information
Health improvement	Standardised mortality ratios, cancer registrations
Fair access	Admission and attendance rates, consultation rates, waiting times
Effective healthcare delivery	% stages of breast cancer at first diagnosis, % surgical procedures considered 'inappropriate'
Efficiency	Costs per healthcare resource group category, practice overheads per list size and number of partners, day case rates
Patient/carer experience	% complaints in various categories, time waiting in outpatients or A&E, consumer surveys (*see* Figure 6.3)
Health outcomes	Psychiatric emergency readmission rates, teenage pregnancy rates, 5-year survival rates for cancers

postoperative infection rates among local trusts and compare with comparable trusts elsewhere.
* The need to understand the scientific evidence, or not, for the efficacy of a particular healthcare intervention.

Drawing on all of these themes, Table 6.2, which is not necessarily comprehensive, summarises some of the main potential sources, issues associated with availability and use for the main information requirements.
   Table 6.2 shows that:

* Many existing information sources and systems are available for PCGs to exploit now. There is a wealth of information about, for example, hospital activity, mortality, prescribing patterns and GMS expenditure, which can be analysed meaningfully at the PCG level.
* In some areas, information may be collected through more ad hoc channels, such as co-ordinating and pooling information from local clinical audit initiatives, and conducting local surveys.
* As *Information for Health* is implemented, over the next few years, new information sources will become available, such as the National Electronic Library for Health and comprehensive 'electronic health records'.

Table 6.2: Information sources and issues associated with usage

Information requirement	Information source	Issues
Budgets and targets associated with individual service agreements	Local plans and allocation process	Budget based on historical activity, moving towards capitation formula. Create spreadsheet of targets to feed monitoring procedures?
Hospital activity levels and financial commitments to date	Trusts	Trust activity data will be routed via NHS-wide clearing service. PCGs will need to agree arrangements for validation, monitoring and systems access with their health authority (HA)
Service quality measures by trust and by service agreement needs	Trust	Need to agree key indicators, consistent with national framework and HA
Profiles of available trust services and associated costs	Trust (via local intranet in future?)	All local PCGs have similar need, so could develop database co-operatively
Referrals by practice	Trust initially (via HA and clearing service); practices later; GP co-operatives for 'out-of-hours' referrals	Uneven coverage and quality of data within practice systems. Better practice data once electronic referral and discharge messaging (national target by year 2002). Routine trust data may only cover admissions. Outpatient data may need more trust attention
Waiting lists and waiting times	Trust, possibly clearing service; waiting times returns	Need to distinguish waiting time for outpatient appointment and inpatient admission. Prospective waiting time (when is next appointment?), cf experience of time waiting (how long did people wait?). Need to review lists of individual long-waiters?
Prescribing patterns by practice/GP	Prescribing and costing data (PACT) via the Prescriptions and Pricing Authority (PPA)	Good quality data, and flexible reporting facilities such as E-PACT being developed. Does not cover hospital-based prescribing
Practice profiles: expenditure and general medical services (GMS) activity levels	Exeter system at the HA	Good quality data. Most HAs have flexible reporting facilities
Population demographics and socioeconomic profiles, deprivation indicators	Office for National Statistics (ONS), census data, local authority (LA), HA, public health common data set (PHCDS), commercial organisations (e.g. CACI)	See below on geography and population statistics. 1991, latest full census year, but LA data more up to date for some aspects

Table 6.2: Continued

Information requirement	Information source	Issues
Mortality and fertility statistics	ONS. Anonymised event-level files, national and local published statistics, including standardised rates, PHCDS	ONS files can be analysed at postcode sector level, and by other geographical groupings which may be approximately mapped to PCGs
Local morbidity patterns	Practice systems; surveys; cancer registrations; local registers, e.g. diabetes; PHCDS; trust data (admissions, outpatients, see above).	See below on Information from primary care and Data quality; most cancers rare at PCG level, so need to pool across years?
Local lifestyle patterns, e.g. smoking, unemployment, housing	Practice systems, LA, local surveys	Many practices routinely collect data on risk factors such as smoking. This might be extracted using tools such as MIQUEST.[5] LA have access to information of housing and other environmental factors
Patient views re demand, service quality	Local surveys, complaints	Survey design needs careful thought and advice from statistician
Measures of outcome / health gain from specific healthcare programmes	Trusts, practices, local clinical audits, local surveys, Exeter system (HA), child health system (immunisation and vaccination) in community trusts	Uneven coverage and quality of data within practice systems is key issue
Evidence of effectiveness of specific interventions	National Electronic Library for Health (once developed), Cochrane Library, Bandolier	Local access to various accredited sources via NHSnet. Access to many non-accredited sources via the Internet
Guidelines and protocols	Local trusts, HA, other PCGs, practices	All local PCGs have similar need, so develop co-operatively? Share using databases on NHSnet/local intranet?
Comparative performance information	HA (local) and Hospital Episodes Statistics (national); common information core; commercial organisations (e.g. CHKS)	Commercial packages and analyses available, e.g. to compare local trust lengths of stay and day case rates by Healthcare Resource Group, with national norms
Verbal and textual communications	Anywhere!	Increasing use of electronic communications
Practice staffing details	Exeter system at HA	

Some key issues

Hospital and community services data coverage

Both Box 6.1 and Table 6.2 reveal important gaps in the coverage of routinely available information. Even for hospital services, where much data collection attention has been focused in the past, some trusts are unable to routinely provide patient-level data sets for activity in outpatients, A&E or for direct access tests such as radiology. For community-based services, there are not only gaps, but fundamental questions about the value of the information currently collected, such as the number of 'face-to-face contacts' for each service. Hospital data coverage will undoubtedly continue to improve. For community, a rethink is needed about what is required and how it is collected. *Information for Health* recognises this, but it will be some time before national solutions are in place. Meanwhile PCGs might consider the costs and benefits of selective collection of simple but more clinically relevant community data.

Statistical analysis

Many of the examples above require comparisons between practices, between PCGs, between trusts and between years. Data often need to be expressed as rates per head of population, which in turn usually need to be standardised – for age and for sex.[8]

Because PCGs are based on populations averaging about 100 000, many conditions of interest may be quite rare. Comparison of small numbers between years, between practices or between PCGs requires extreme caution and sound statistical advice. It may be necessary to pool information across PCGs to investigate time trends, or across years to investigate practice variations.

Geography

Most PCGs do not follow exact geographic boundaries, but are defined by practice populations. Many patients of a PCG may fall outside the geographic limits of the health authority to whom the PCG is accountable. This poses a problem when much of the routine comparative information is based on standard populations related to local authority boundaries, wards, enumeration districts or is linked to postcodes. Some approximate solutions will need to be developed, with 'fuzzy' matching of postcode-defined areas and practice catchment areas.

Population statistics

The apparently simple question 'What is the resident population of our PCG?' does not have a simple answer. First it depends on whether an aggregation of practice-based or some geographically based estimates is used. The former relates better to the PCG reality, but suffers from important exclusions (non-registered individuals) and false inclusions ('ghost' patients). The second suffers from the problem of geography (see above) but has the advantages of being widely used by The Department of Health, health authorities and local authorities. These official estimates seek to allow for issues such as homeless people, students and other temporary residents. As well as population estimates, population projections are produced, with obvious value in forecasting and planning. But there is a second problem – estimates and projections used within the NHS do not necessarily tally well with those used within local authorities.

When calculating rates it is essential to ensure that the numerator (e.g. number of deaths) and the denominator (i.e. the population size) actually do relate to the same population. PCGs will need to work closely with population experts within the local authority, the health authority and elsewhere to ensure sensible common approaches.

Information from primary care

Practice systems are the great untapped information resource of the NHS. As practices record more and more clinical information on their systems, the value of the data to PCGs increases. Unfortunately, there are some fairly challenging problems to address before morbidity data can simply be routinely sent down the line to the PCG, as trials of the MIQUEST software have shown.[5] Problems include the following:

- Even within a practice there is great variation in how much clinical information is recorded, so there are gaps in data coverage.
- The different types of practice systems record and store information in different ways, so there are data inconsistencies.
- Even when clinical coding standards such as the Read codes[4] are used, they can be applied in different ways in different practices, or even within practices, making comparisons difficult.

Practice systems can no longer be considered as isolated, and PCG developments will put greater emphasis on the need to intercommunicate and share. Having connectivity through the NHSnet will not be enough, however. These systems need to develop within a framework of standards covering technical areas (e.g. networking protocols), confidentiality and security standards, as well as protocols for data collection and coding.

Adopting national standards[9] is an important prerequisite for greater information sharing and electronic communications among practices and PCGs. PCGs have a key role in promoting standards and encouraging standardised clinical data recording and coding across their practices.

Data quality

Routine data from trusts and from primary care is currently far from perfect in terms of its coverage, completeness and consistency. The history of data collection in the NHS has been to strive for 100% coverage of 100% accurate data, and to fail! So considerable resources are expended, yet the data are rubbished and underused. PCGs will need to consider the trade-offs between data quality and effort, recognising that often 'the best is the enemy of the good'! Data should normally flow from routine operation procedures. Where it doesn't, additional data collection has an additional cost.

PCGs have an important role in encouraging and enforcing greater data quality within both primary and secondary care. PCGs may include data quality clauses in their service agreements, and may possibly undertake selective systematic data quality audits.

Access and tools

Although PCGs will be information-hungry, they will not necessarily need to collect and store much new information for themselves. The main requirement is to gain access to databases held by the health authority or the trusts, within practices or nationally. The next section discusses the role of NHSnet in this.

PCGs will also require simple tools to allow these various data to be interrogated, manipulated and presented in flexible ways. Some tools such as Electronic-PACT or health authority executive information systems may already exist. Others will need to be developed using, for example, standard spreadsheet software.

Communications

PCGs will not be working in isolation. Indeed their very composition reflects the multiprofessional, multiagency nature of their remit. Therefore two-way sharing of information and communicating with a wide range of other organisations is not an option. The likely volume of communications means it will need to be easy, cheap and effective.

Types of communication?

We can think of the communication needs of PCGs under three broad headings.

Person to person

If we want to share information with another individual or group of individuals, we might choose to meet with them face to face, or to phone or fax them. Increasingly e-mail, electronic forums and electronic distribution of documents will be seen as more efficient communication modes for sharing notes of meetings, holding virtual meetings or consulting with colleagues.

Person to computer

Examples of this might include:

- Browsing the NHS intranet, known as NHSnet, to access websites containing information on the evidence for and against a particular healthcare intervention.
- Accessing a database held within the local trust to look up the time of the next available slot for an ENT appointment.
- Examining the latest local population projections produced by the local authority, available via a local 'intranet'.

The intelligence model, above, implies that much information will be 'browsed' rather than held locally. There is tremendous value, in terms of consistency, quality and efficiency, in holding and maintaining common information once centrally for all to access, rather than in a myriad of locations and formats. For example, local demographic statistics or local clinical protocols and guidelines could be maintained by an agreed data custodian for all local PCGs, the health authority and the trusts, accessed through user-friendly, web-browsing technology and interrogation tools.

Computer to computer

In this case, information is automatically sent from one system, received and integrated into the database of another, without the need for (too much!) human intervention. An example of this electronic data interchange (EDI) might be the routine extraction of anonymised activity data from each practice system into a PCG morbidity database. Information would be extracted and sent in a predefined format, using standard codes.

NHSnet will become a key medium for communication amongst NHS organisations over the next few years, supporting all three types of communication. There is central funding to allow all general practices to connect to NHSnet, and it is the only approved, secure network for exchanging confidential patient data within the NHS.[1]

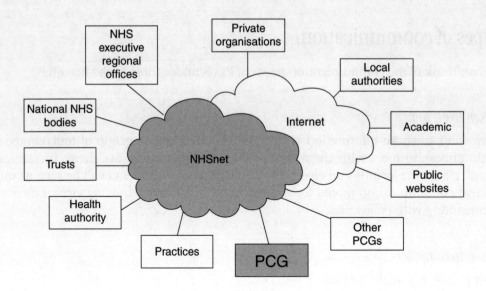

Figure 6.5: Most organisations with whom the PCG communicates will be connected to NHSnet directly or indirectly.

Figure 6.5 shows how the NHS will also be able to access information from non-NHS organisations, via a secure gateway to the global Internet. Most practices, trusts and health authorities are likely to be connected to NHSnet before the end of 1999.

Challenges regarding communications

For the next few years at least, not all GPs or all hospital consultants, for example, will have access to NHSnet from their desktop computer. Indeed, outside of general practice, many clinicians still do not have access to any computer terminal. In many cases, further investment will be needed in local area networks and compatible software for e-mail. There are also issues concerning the relative merits of NHSnet versus the Internet for certain types of communication, and about the practicalities of implementing security policies.

It is likely to be some time, therefore, until the full potential of electronic communications can be exploited, but PCGs should be in the driving seat and can achieve some early benefits. PCGs have a potentially important role in helping their practices to take a co-ordinated approach and obtain early benefits.

Concluding remarks

The demanding new roles of PCGs must be mediated through the sensible use of information and communications technologies. The diversity of information, its sources and its applications means that there isn't a single 'PCG system' waiting to be developed. This overview highlights some of the areas where progress can be made now, but it also sets out a fairly challenging agenda for the future. Clearly it will take some time – years not months – for many of the requirements to be realised. For many reasons a pragmatic, incremental, evolutionary approach will be required.[10] This means that PCGs should:

- start simply, exploiting what is available now
- maximise the opportunities for co-operating and sharing
- find ways of collecting new information where there is an important gap
- give an early priority to investment in a communications infrastructure which will provide short-term benefits as well as supporting strategic developments
- minimise transaction costs associated with the 'control' functions
- seek expert advice.

On the last point, the wide range of information requirements and analyses outlined above implies fairly well-developed information knowledge and skills at PCG-level. PCGs need a good level of awareness of the sources of information, and the strengths and weaknesses of different information, access to statistical, analytical and presentational skills, and occasional support for the design and analysis of surveys.

Individual PCGs will need to decide how best to meet these needs – by employing and training appropriate PCG staff, by pooling resources and sharing across PCGs, or through service level agreements with another NHS or commercial organisation. In the early years, there is likely to be a heavy dependence upon health authority information, library and public health departments. Similarly, the heavy reliance on information technology (IT) and communications technology will mean that all PCG staff will need a minimum level of IT literacy. Training and development in these areas must be given a high priority in the early years.

References

1 NHS Executive (1998) *Information for Health. An Information Strategy for the Modern NHS.* NHSE, London.

2 Healthcare Resource Groups (1995) *National Statistics 1994/5. Acute Care 95.* CHKS, London.

3 Health Services Research Unit (1996) *The UK SF-36: analysis and interpretation manual.* HSRU, Oxford.

4 NHS Executive (1996) *Read Codes in Use.* NHSE, London.

5   NHS Executive (1996) *Collection of Health Data from General Practice: overview.* NHSE, London.

6   NHS Executive (1998) *The New NHS Modern and Dependable. A National Framework for Assessing Performance Consultation Document.* NHSE, London.

7   NHS Executive (1998) *A First Class Service; Quality in the new NHS.* NHSE, London.

8   Alderson M (1983) *An Introduction to Epidemiology* (2e). Macmillan Press, Basingstoke.

9   NHS Executive (1998) *Requirements for Accreditation for Practice Systems* (Version 4). NHSE, London.

10 NHS Executive (1998) *The New NHS Modern and Dependable. Developing Primary Care Groups.* HSC 1998/139. NHSE, London.

CHAPTER SEVEN

Clinical governance

John Derry

What does clinical governance mean?

The concept of clinical governance was first introduced in the White Paper *The New NHS: modern, dependable*, published in December 1997.[1] It is defined in the consultation document *A First Class Service. Quality in the New NHS*[2] as 'a framework through which NHS organisations are accountable for continuously improving the quality of their services and safeguarding high standards of care by creating an environment in which excellence in clinical care will flourish'. An underlying principle is to parallel the concept of corporate governance[3] (ensuring sound business and financial management), giving equal weight to the quality of clinical care provided by the organisation. In this way the responsibility for quality of clinical care is shared between clinicians and managers: clinical quality is not solely the preserve of clinicians, but 'quality is everybody's business'. It is important to see this shared responsibility as a two-way process. Clinicians may at first be concerned about managers looking at the quality of clinical care, but equally managers must now consider the effects of their decisions on clinical quality. Two further quotes from *A First Class Service* underline these points:

- 'The principles of clinical governance apply to all those who provide or manage patient care services in the NHS.'
- 'For the first time, the NHS will be required to adopt a structured and coherent approach to clinical quality, placing duties and expectations on local health care organisations as well as individuals.'

A First Class Service places clinical governance at the centre of a system for continuous quality improvement in the NHS. In it the wider context of setting, delivering and monitoring quality standards is described and the concept of clinical governance is explored in more depth. The clinical governance framework is intended to strengthen existing systems for quality control, based on clinical standards, evidence-based practice and learning the lessons of poor performance. Four strands of work within the framework are described:

- identify and build on good practice
- assess and minimise the risk of untoward events
- investigate problems as these arise and ensure lessons are learnt
- support health professionals in delivering quality care.

From these, five essential building blocks for the work of clinical governance can be identified:

- clinical audit
- clinical effectiveness
- risk management
- quality assurance
- development of staff and organisations.

These already exist to varying degrees in many sectors of primary care but have tended to operate in separate compartments. What is new about clinical governance is that it brings these building blocks together into an integrated system for improving quality of care. If clinical governance is to be effective in producing lasting change it must be acceptable to all those who work in primary care, which requires that the building blocks must be placed on the right foundations.

Development of clinical governance in the NHS requires establishment of the right culture and leadership[4] and this applies as much to primary care as NHS trusts and health authorities. Clinicians and managers will need to work in an open partnership together, sharing ideas and good practice, and valuing education, research and lifelong learning. Users of health services and their carers will need to be fully involved in this partnership. The tendency to blame individuals when things go wrong must be replaced with an approach that recognises that virtually everyone in the NHS is striving to do the best they can and looks for faults in systems of care which can be learned from and remedied.

Implications for primary care groups – NHSE guidance

The Health Service Circular *Developing Primary Care Groups*[5] provides more detail about the implementation of clinical governance in primary care.

> *Each PCG must also appoint a senior doctor or nurse to take responsibility at board level to ensure that a proper process for Clinical Governance is in place. That person will take responsibility for formulation of an agreed action plan. Each practice within the PCG will also wish to ensure that one person is remitted to take forward the plan.*

The Annual Accountability Agreement between primary care group (PCG) and health authority will include reports on action taken under the principles of clinical governance. Section 3 of the supporting guidance to this HSC sets out the clinical governance arrangements for PCGs.

In this guidance, emphasis is placed on achievable change, focusing on specific issues, and a process of clinical governance that is reflective and supportive for doctors, nurses and other health professions operating within PCGs. Attention is drawn to the need to involve key stakeholders, especially patients, at an early stage. In recognition of the fact that clinical governance needs to be developed from the ground up rather than imposed in order to be truly effective, the guidance suggests that PCGs should apply the principles of clinical governance to only two areas in the first year. One should be chosen from four topics of national importance:

- antibiotic prescribing
- cancer services
- mental health services
- coronary heart disease.

The other should be an area of local concern that fits in with the Health Improvement Programme (HImP). For example, addressing the healthcare needs of a particular patient group, or the organisation and standards for delivery of a particular service provided within the PCG. Detailed information about the four national priority areas is contained in *National Service Frameworks for Coronary Heart Disease and Mental Health Services*, which are to be published in spring 1999, the 1994 Calman-Hine report on cancer services and in the report from the Standing Medical Advisory Committee on antibiotic prescribing, *The Path of Least Resistance*[6] published in September 1998.

Developing clinical governance at PCG-level

Although a senior doctor or nurse will take primary responsibility for developing the processes of clinical governance on behalf of the PCG Board, the whole Board is accountable through its Chair to the Chief Executive of the health authority for the operation of the PCG. It is essential that the Board supports the clinical governance lead by sharing responsibility and avoiding the isolation of quality from day-to-day operations. In this way the PCG Board will provide essential leadership, demonstrating to all the constituents of the PCG how clinical governance is everyone's responsibility and duty.

The clinical governance lead

The clinical governance lead will need to develop effective working relationships with general practices and the other providers of primary healthcare services in the PCG. Each practice within the PCG will need to identify one person to implement the PCG action plan for developing clinical governance[7] and it may be helpful for these practice leads to form a PCG clinical governance working group, chaired by the PCG lead.

Establishing the right culture for clinical governance throughout the constituents of the PCG will be a major concern of the clinical governance lead and will require good leadership skills. The lead will need to maintain the trust and respect of colleagues in practices by demonstrating that information about the quality of care being provided is used as an opportunity for learning and improvement rather than criticism and blame. The underlying philosophy must be that lapses in quality are usually due to faults in the systems of providing care rather than inadequacies of any individual.

The PCG action plan for clinical governance

Responsibility for formulation of the PCG action plan will be taken by the clinical governance lead. The plan should be developed with help from local experts in national, clinical and practice audit, postgraduate education and training, evidence-based care and organisation development, but national guidance makes it clear that the action plan should remain under the direction of and firmly owned by the members of the PCG.[8] Also emphasised is the need to involve key stakeholders, especially patients, at an early stage of developing the plan. PCGs are expected to work together to share ideas, learning and special expertise. It may well be helpful for the PCG clinical governance leads within a health authority to have a forum in which to meet together to pool ideas and resources. Existing primary care audit groups (MAAGs and their successors) are often well placed to fulfil this function, though will need further development to become clinical governance support groups. Effective integration of GP tutors and others involved in primary care education will be essential.

The action plan will need to set out the changes needed throughout the PCG to develop clinical governance principles for the chosen priority topics. An important first step will be some assessment of the level of development in individual practices of the components of clinical governance. Information about current activity and performance in the priority areas will need to be collected and collated. Plans for development will need to address the specific barriers to the changes desired with a combination of different interventions tailored to individual situations[9] (see also the section on Implementing change).

As is recognised in Health Service Circular 1998/139,[5] not everything that needs to be done in developing clinical governance can be tackled at once. In many respects the progress made towards establishing a comprehensive framework for clinical governance is more important than the starting point. PCGs and individual practices will vary in the degree to which the parts of clinical governance are already in place. PCGs with minimal devolved responsibility will not be expected to have as comprehensive clinical governance processes as those in a primary care trust or other NHS trust. Progress of a PCG towards trust status and independence will require development of clinical governance procedures as comprehensive as those in any NHS trust organisation.

The components of clinical governance for a PCG

The description of clinical governance in an NHS trust can be used as a starting point to explore what the components of clinical governance might be for a primary care trust. This can then form a model on which to base development of clinical governance in PCGs and general practices within a PCG. The British Association of Medical Managers (BAMM) has produced a useful checklist for assessing the development of clinical governance within a trust[10] and this is used in Table 7.1 to describe what clinical governance might look like in a PCG. The functions of PCGs as providers of primary care and commissioners of other healthcare services are dealt with separately in the table as they require different clinical governance systems. It must be emphasised that Table 7.1 represents a description of fully developed clinical governance in a PCG approaching primary care trust status. It will take several years to develop these processes in many PCGs.

Table 7.1:   Clinical governance systems in a PCG

System	PCG as provider	PCG as commissioner
Quality improvement processes – clinical audit – integrated into organisational quality programme	Inter-practice clinical audit of agreed priority areas with feedback of comparative results. Audit results inform learning and development plans	Referrals audit informs commissioning plans. Seeks evidence of clinical audit activity relevant to HImP in reports from trusts
Leadership skills developed at clinical team level	PCG lead has effective working relationships with other Board members and practice leads. Clear statement of PCG priorities and establishing 'no blame' culture	Seeks evidence of appropriate culture and clear leadership in trusts, including defined clinical team structure
Evidence-based practice and infrastructure in place and used	Access to electronic information databases. Training for critical appraisal, finding evidence, etc. Implementation of evidence-based guidelines	Uses evidence to inform commissioning plans. Asks trusts about their evidence-based practice infrastructure and training
Clinical risk reduction programmes in place and of high quality	Monitors and promotes establishment of these in practices	Asks trusts to outline their programmes, including examples of action plans
Adverse events – detected, investigated and lessons learnt translated into change in practice	Monitors and promotes establishment of systems in practices to detect 'near misses' and review premature deaths, etc.	Asks trusts to outline their programmes, seeking evidence of changes
Systematic learning from clinical complaints, with translation into change in practice	Receives regular reports from practices reviewing complaints, identifying and responding to common themes	Asks trusts to outline their programmes, seeking evidence of changes

Table 7.1:   Continued

System	PCG as provider	PCG as commissioner
Poor clinical performance identified early and dealt with skill, speed and sensitivity to avoid harm to patients	Explicit commitment to professional standards (e.g. GMC, UKCC). Explicit policy for dealing with concerns, including named individuals to be contacted by any individual working in the PCG and practices. Links to systems of local professional self-regulation and existing procedures, e.g. LMC, health authority panels. Ensures that all clinical staff participate in clinical audit	Asks trusts to describe their procedures. Has explicit policy for acting on concerns about trust staff
Continuing professional development (CPD) programmes in place, reflecting principles of clinical governance	Reviews practices' CPD programmes and has overall PCG CPD programme built upon assessment of practice needs. CPD linked to implementation of PCG development priorities, including HImP	Asks trusts to report on their CPD programmes, assessing relevance to HImP, links to clinical audit and risk management programmes, etc.
Quality of data for monitoring clinical care is of consistently high standard	Collects routine data from practices and feeds back results of quality checks. Agreed policies for clinical term coding, clinical record-keeping. Data collection linked to performance monitoring requirements. Provides training for practices on importance of data quality, correct use of clinical coding and computer systems, etc.	Receives reports from trusts about data quality assurance system in place. Regularly reviews and validates practices' referral data

An alternative perspective of clinical governance has been provided by Pat Oakley, Director of Practices made Perfect, at a series of workshops for NHS staff held by the Anglia and Oxford Region NHS Executive during 1998 (*see* Table 7.2). A clinical governance policy and management framework is based around a whole-systems approach to quality assurance as developed in other industries and underpinned by the regulatory and legal duties imposed on NHS organisations. This framework has three dimensions, each with several components.

Importantly, this framework integrates non-clinical risk management imperatives with clinical governance requirements. Inquiries in both the NHS and in other industries following major disasters and serious incidents have highlighted the need for a systematic whole-systems approach to the management of complex organisations to prevent 'disasters waiting to happen'.

Table 7.2:   Policy and management framework for clinical governance

Safe organisational practices	• a safe environment for work • staff recruitment and retention practices • Health and Safety at work policies • Employment Law followed
Healthy staff who are fit to practice	• psychological health of workforce • dealing with harassment and bullying • effective teams and teamworking • support for individuals (professional, managerial, pastoral)
Safe, up-to-date practices	• effective clinical and care practices (EBP) • changing practice (audit and peer review, complaints procedures, attitudes and behaviours) • staffing numbers and skill mix

Clinical governance at practice level

The BAMM checklist for clinical governance can also be used to outline what might be the elements of clinical governance in a general practice or primary healthcare team. As before, this description is comprehensive and many practices will take several years to develop all of these elements. In addition, it may well be inappropriate for smaller practices to operate all of the systems described. Table 7.3 sets out suggested components of clinical governance in a general practice.

Table 7.3:   Systems of clinical governance in a general practice

System	General practice functions
Quality improvement processes – clinical audit – integrated into organisational quality programme	Participates in PCG inter-practice audit programme. Multidisciplinary clinical audit also carried out according to Practice Development Plan. Results used to inform CPD in practice
Leadership skills developed at clinical team level	PCG lead has effective working relationships with whole practice team. Leaders identified for nursing team(s). Regular practice meetings – ?multidisciplinary quality team – to review quality development. Evidence of 'no blame' culture and systems approach to problem solving
Evidence-based practice and infrastructure in place and used	Attended training for critical appraisal, finding evidence, etc. Access to electronic information databases and secondary sources of appraised evidence (journals, etc.). Implementing evidence-based guidelines, including audit based on best evidence
Clinical risk reduction programmes in place and of high quality	E.g. regular review of repeat prescribing system; audit of anticoagulation control; audit of minor surgery; logging of telephone contacts from patients

Table 7.3: Continued

System	General practice functions
Adverse events – detected, investigated and lessons learnt translated into change in practice	Systems to identify and report 'near misses' and other adverse events. Reviews of these to identify learning points and change systems accordingly. Culture that cherishes 'near misses' as opportunity for learning
Systematic learning from clinical complaints, with translation into change in practice	Regular review of 'in-house' complaints to identify common themes and trends; appropriate changes made as needed
Poor clinical performance identified early and dealt with skill, speed and sensitivity to avoid harm to patients	Explicit commitment to professional standards (e.g. GMC, UKCC). Explicit policy for dealing with concerns, including named individuals to be contacted by any individual working in the practice. Knowledge of systems of local professional self-regulation (currently under development), also existing procedures, e.g. LMC, health authority panels. All clinical staff participate in peer review and clinical audit programmes
CPD programmes in place, reflecting principles of clinical governance	Practice CPD programme reported to PCG, identifying items linked to PCG priorities. Individuals' CPD programmes relate to practice and PCG development plans. Staff and doctor appraisal systems in operation. Results of clinical audit used to identify CPD needs
Quality of data for monitoring clinical care is of consistently high standard	Policies for routine data collection, including agreed clinical term coding, recording of clinical contacts. Regular reviews of data quality. Attends training on correct use of clinical coding and computer systems, etc. Validates referral data from PCG

Difficulties for clinical governance in PCGs

An important organisational difference between a PCG and a NHS trust that affects clinical governance is the different contractual arrangements for individuals providing healthcare within a PCG. In a trust, virtually everyone working for the trust is an employee of the trust, whereas a PCG covers many different groups of healthcare providers (family doctors, community nurses, health visitors, midwives, dentists, pharmacists, optometrists, ophthalmic medical practitioners, chiropodists, podiatrists, physiotherapists, occupational therapists, etc.) with several employment arrangements. Some are self-employed (e.g. GPs, dentists), some are employees of NHS trusts (e.g. community midwives, district nurses, health visitors) and some are employed by GPs (e.g. practice nurses). Others are employed by non-NHS businesses (e.g. pharmacists, optometrists). Those working for NHS trusts will be subject to the clinical governance arrangements of their employing trust, but may also need to work within the clinical governance systems of the PCG. Quite how clinical governance might operate for those working in non-NHS organisations remains to be seen.

A further complicating factor for PCGs is that individuals will be working in several sites, with differing sizes of team and working environment, spread over a geographical area. This will affect the implementation of clinical governance at individual and team level and will require the PCG, and particularly the clinical governance lead, to develop a good understanding of the particular circumstances pertaining in each functional unit.

NHS trust employees working within a PCG (e.g. community midwives, district nurses, health visitors) may face problems because of working under two systems of clinical governance – the trust's and the PCG's. This potential difficulty is most likely to occur for activities which cross the interface between PCG and trust responsibilities, such as child protection procedures or obstetric risk management. PCGs and trusts will need to develop their clinical governance systems in these areas in ways that take this dual accountability into consideration. In many cases the trust systems are likely to be more established than those of the PCG and PCG leads will be able to build the PCG clinical governance procedures on those of the trust. An important principle must be that the clinical governance systems of either organisation must not interfere with the effective operation of local clinical teams and teamworking.

Implementing change – how to develop clinical governance

Having developed an understanding of what clinical governance means for PCGs, set out the vision of what is to be achieved and what it might look like when fully established, the challenge is to make it happen.

An excellent review of the theory and practice of implementing change in the general practice setting was published in 1992 by Richard Grol.[11] He describes four steps for dissemination and implementation of good practice each of which may be attended by specific problems or barriers (Table 7.4). These barriers may exist because of characteristics of either the individual practitioner whose behaviour needs to change, or the organisation in which he or she works – the practice setting.

Barriers within the individual practitioner can be in competence, motivation and attitude, and personal characteristics such as age, experience, learning style, self-confidence and willingness to change. Barriers that may exist in the practice setting can be social factors and structural, logistic and organisational factors.

Recognition of these many different barriers and factors which may impede change leads to the understanding that a variety and combination of methods is needed to implement good practice successfully. Methods used should be directed towards existing barriers and problems with implementation and carried out at several levels, e.g. at PCG, practice and individual clinician levels. Different methods have been shown to have different effectiveness at different levels. There is a growing body of literature around the implementation of change and research evidence from controlled trials is being synthesised

Table 7.4: Steps and barriers in implementing new guidelines – for example, the implementation of an antibiotic prescribing policy in a PCG (adapted from Grol[11])

Steps	Features	Barriers and problems	Example barriers	Example solutions
Orientation	Attention and becoming informed about the existence of new guidelines Feeling interest, commitment	No reading or selective reading No continuing professional development No contact with colleagues No needs or interest	Lack of locally provided medical education An isolated, single-handed GP	PCG organises locally based study day on new antibiotic prescribing policy and organises locum cover to allow single-handed GPs to attend
Insight	Understanding the guidelines Awareness of (gaps in) own performance Persuasion of the need to change	Insufficient knowledge or skills No awareness of gaps in own routines Not participating in clinical audit Overestimation of own performance	GPs don't have information about their own antibiotic prescribing behaviour and don't accept there is any need to change	PCG produces and circulates information from PACT data comparing antibiotic prescribing costs and volumes, for different practices and for individual GPs
Acceptance	Positive attitude to the new guidelines Intention to change Confidence in success	Seeing more disadvantages than advantages Change not seen as feasible Not feeling involved, committed Expecting problems, negative consequences Negative attitude of opinion leaders Change requires extra time or money	GPs worried that patients expect to be given antibiotics and that explaining new policy will take up more consulting time	PCG produces patient information leaflets for common self-limiting minor ailments, explaining why antibiotics not needed PCG involves local community pharmacists in reinforcing policy and educating patients about appropriate use of antibiotics
Change	Actual implementation in practice Experimentation Recognition of positive outcomes Maintenance of change	Seeing no concrete alternatives Inadequate practice premises No confidence in success Forgetting, reverting to old routines Negative outcomes of change No reinforcement	GPs lapse back into old patterns of prescribing Some GPs complain that a number of patients keep coming back for antibiotic prescriptions	PCG provides regular comparative reports about antibiotic prescribing from quarterly PACT data PCG summarises evidence from GP research that not giving antibiotics for sore throats reduces patients' intention to consult in the future

into systematic reviews of the effectiveness of different interventions at changing the behaviour of clinicians,[12–17] particularly by members of the Cochrane Collaboration Effective Practice and Organisation of Care Group. Table 7.5 summarises the research evidence for different kinds of intervention designed to change practice in a primary care setting.

Table 7.5: Effectiveness of interventions designed to change practice in primary care (from Grol[11])

	Intervention	Effect
Facilitating, educational methods	Mailed educational materials, journals, mass media	–
	Continuing medical education, group learning, courses, tutorials	+/–
	Face-to-face education, individual instruction	+
	Audit and feedback (by computer)	+/–
	Reminders (by computer)	+
	Peer reviews, quality circles, practice visiting	+
	Patient influence	?
	Structural arrangements (provisions, staff)	?
	Barriers to stop unwanted activity	+/–
Coercive, controlling methods	Incentives or sanctions	+/–
	Rules, laws, obligations, certifications, contracts	?

References

1   Secretary of State for Health (1997) *The New NHS: modern, dependable.* Stationery Office, London.

2   NHS Executive (1998) *A First Class Service; Quality in the New NHS.* NHSE, London.

3   *Report of the Committee on Financial Aspects of Corporate Governance* (1992) Gee, London.

4   Scally G, Donaldson LJ (1998) Clinical governance and the drive for quality improvement in the new NHS in England. *BMJ.* **317**: 61–5.

5   NHS Executive (1998) *Developing Primary Care Groups.* HSC 1998/139. NHSE, London.

6   Standing Medical Advisory Committee (1998) *The Path of Least Resistance.* Standing Medical Advisory Committee, London.

7   NHS Executive (1998) *Developing Primary Care Groups.* HSC 1998/139. Para. 106.

8   NHS Executive (1998) *Developing Primary Care Groups.* HSC 1998/139. Para. 106–8.

9   Grol R (1997) Beliefs and evidence in changing clinical practice. *BMJ.* **315**: 418–21.

10   British Association of Medical Managers (1998) *Clinical Governance in the New NHS.* BAMM, Stockport.

11   Grol R (1992) Implementing guidelines in general practice care. *Quality in Health Care.* **1**: 184–91.

12 Oxman AD, Thomson MA, Davis DA et al. (1995) No magic bullets: a systematic review of 102 trials of interventions to improve professional practice. *Canandian Medical Association Journal.* **153**: 1423–31.

13 Thomson MA, Oxman AD, Davis DA et al. (1997) Audit and feedback to improve health professional practice and health care outcomes (Part I) (Cochrane Review). In: *The Cochrane Library, Issue 4, 1998.* Update Software, Oxford.

14 Thomson MA, Oxman AD, Davis DA et al. (1997) Audit and feedback to improve health professional practice and health care outcomes (Part II) (Cochrane Review). In: *The Cochrane Library, Issue 4, 1998.* Update Software, Oxford.

15 Thomson MA, Oxman AD, Haynes RB et al. (1997) Local opinion leaders to improve health professional practice and health care outcomes (Cochrane Review). In: *The Cochrane Library, Issue 4, 1998.* Update Software, Oxford.

16 Thomson MA, Oxman AD, Davis DA et al. (1997) Outreach visits to improve health professional practice and health care outcomes (Cochrane Review). In: *The Cochrane Library, Issue 4, 1998.* Update Software, Oxford.

17 Freemantle N, Harvey EL, Wolf F et al. (1997) Printed educational materials to improve the behaviour of health care professionals and patient outcomes (Cochrane Review). In: *The Cochrane Library, Issue 4, 1998.* Update Software, Oxford.

Further reading

Risk management

NHS Executive (1993) *Risk management in the NHS.* EL(93)111. NHSE, London.

Vincent C (1997) Risk, safety, and the darker side of quality. *BMJ.* **314**: 1775.

Vincent C (ed.) (1996) *Clinical Risk Management.* BMJ, London.

Professional self-regulation

General Medical Council (1998) *Good Medical Practice.* GMC, London.

Significant event audit

Pringle M, Bradley C (1994) Significant event auditing: a user's guide. *Audit Trends.* **2**: 20–3.

Pringle M, Bradley C, Carmichael C et al. (1995) *Significant event auditing.* (Occasional Paper 70) Royal College of General Practitioners, London.

Clinical audit

Fraser RC, Lakhani MK, Baker RH (eds) (1998) *Evidence-based Audit in General Practice: from principles to practice.* Butterworth-Heinemann, Oxford.

Irvine D, Irvine S (eds) (1991) *Making Sense of Audit.* Radcliffe Medical Press, Oxford.

Marinker M (ed.) (1990) *Medical Audit and General Practice.* BMJ, London.

CHAPTER EIGHT

Implications for primary care

John Rawlinson

Introduction

Primary care groups (PCGs) are set to have the single most important effect on the development of primary care since it began. Evolution, not revolution is the message from the Department of Health on the new NHS. The evolution, however, appears to be more revolution by stealth.

This chapter reviews the potential effects on primary care development, looking initially at the present situation, with some explanation of organisational structure. The areas of development that will be affected by PCG formation are then reviewed, using specific examples to illustrate areas of change that are particularly likely and challenging. Finally the impact on future development is reviewed, with some possible scenarios for the future.

The aim in this chapter is to stimulate debate at PCG-level on looking at the ways primary care can be developed, as well as the potential hindrances along this developmental path.

Up until April 1999, GPs in primary care who were not part of one of the Primary Care Act pilot schemes were, in the main, independent (contractors) who had a contract with the health authority to provide general medical services (GMS). They may have been in a fundholding practice where, for up to the previous 8 years, they had been trying to achieve the best for their patients at a practice level. They may have been part of a commissioning group, acting on behalf of a group of practices to obtain the best, but without any direct financial power. Other commissioning arrangements included multi-funds, total purchasing pilots (TPPs), locality planning and Primary Care Act pilots. From 1 April, there will be fundamental differences from what has gone on before. Every GP practice will become part of a PCG, there is no opt out clause – collaboration and co-operation are the new disciplines – not only between practices, but between primary care teams, the health authority, trusts, local authority and the public. Primary care boards will be accountable to the health authority at all levels.

Old situation

General practitioners

GPs are independent contractors who may work together in varying numbers to run small businesses (the business is general practice). They usually work from surgeries, which are built or adapted for the purpose of providing primary care services to a registered population within their locality.

Staff

GPs employ staff who are accountable to them, and GPs are responsible for ensuring that the employment rights, health and safety at work and a healthy working environment for their staff are fulfilled.

Funding

The budget for all activities in the practice (e.g. premises, staff, computers, prescribing) comes from the centre devolved down to health authorities, who are responsible for ensuring equitable distribution of general medical services cash limited (GMSCL) funds in a fair and equitable way to all practices in their area. Occasionally formulae are used to decide on fair distribution (e.g. the budget for staff may be based on the number of GPs, patients, branch surgeries and deprivation).

From 1 April 1999, PCGs have a role to play in the distribution of some of the monies going to practices. To understand the implications for primary care development, we need to look at the change in responsibility of this fund distribution (*see* Figures 8.1 and 8.2).

New message

The new message for PCGs on the distribution of funds to practices is that there will be more local sensitivity. With this comes both opportunities and threats. Devolution of responsibility for setting staff reimbursement and computer reimbursement at PCG level could provide the opportunity for a fairer and more equitable share out. If we assume that health authorities have developed a formula for distribution of these funds and that this has not always led to a full uptake of funds, then it is possible for PCGs to be more reactive to their practice needs. This is illustrated in the example in Box 8.1.

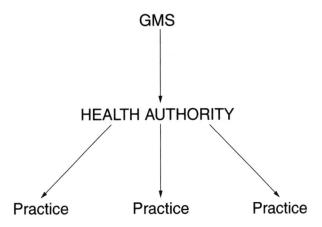

Figure 8.1: Existing fund distribution.

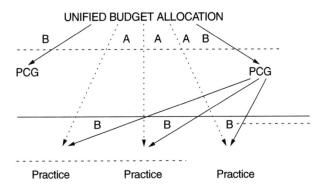

Guaranteed floor for total GMSCL at present allocation plus uplift for inflation.

Total = A (premises and computer capital costs)
      Payment passes direct to practice
    = B (staff costs and computer maintenance)
      Payments are handled by the PCG

Guaranteed subfloor at PCG level for B payments (staff costs and computer maintenance)

Exisiting Red Book provisions at practice level with one year's notice of any change as well as current Red Book protection.

Figure 8.2: New PCG fund distribution. GMS cash limited funds within a unified budget.

Box 8.1:   Resource allocation

Acceptable model
Each practice in capitation model:
Practice A has funds of £50 000
Practice B has funds of £30 000
Practice A uses up £45 000
Practice B development could use £5000
Solution: Practice B receives £5000 from Practice A budget.

Unacceptable model
Each practice in capitation model:
Practice A has funds of £50 000
Practice B has funds of £30 000
Practice A uses up funds of £55 000
Practice B uses up funds of £25 000

The problem is that Practice A would have to make redundancies for Practice B to utilise its extra allocation of £5000. However, there is still inequity between the two practices. How will the PCG deal with Practice A which is 'overspending'? What will the relationship be between Practice A and Practice B when Practice B might perceive that Practice A is using up Practice B's budget?

Role of the PCG Board

The role of the Board, in particular the Chief Executive Officer, will be essential in negotiating a settlement between various practices when it comes to resource allocation disputes. This may be the most important aspect of the Chief Executive's role in the first year. Further, the Chair of the PCG Board will need considerable skill, especially if his or her own practice is involved in a dispute. The Board would be well advised to decide upon the principles of budget allocation before any figures for practices are applied. Because the PCG will be a subcommittee of the health authority, any solution will have to be acceptable to their Chief Executive.

Pace of change

Budget reallocations involving practices having to relinquish funds currently being used for established activities will need careful timing: slow enough to allow any practice losing funds (especially if redundancy is involved) adequate time for change, but rapid enough to be meaningful. There may be the need for an honest broker (e.g. the local medical committee) to help PCGs manage the potential conflicts between practices so that there is not a breakdown in the new working arrangements. Practices may be able to manage these changes by natural wastage, redistribution of staff, changes in working practice and, finally, if absolutely necessary, by redundancy.

Ring-fencing

It is worth remembering that GMS cash limited monies have been protected by a one-way valve to ensure the funding of general practice. The opportunities are there to expand the role played at primary care level by the transference of services (and hence funds) from secondary care, while there is no shift in the opposite direction.

Shared resources

With the unification of budgets, the opportunity for PCGs to share resources of certain administrative details could lead to significant cost savings. These could be reinvested in practices for development of other areas, initially within their own envelope, or if the PCG felt appropriate, in other areas relating to primary care.

Box 8.2:   Examples of resource sharing in PCGs

Practice-based activities likely to remain individual
- Consultations
- Nursing
- Reception

Practice-based activities that offer possibility of sharing
- Payroll systems
- Bulk ordering
    - practice essentials
    - computers
- Shared computer hardware/maintenance contracts
- PCG intranet
- Practice management across practices
- Assistants/salaried general practitioners

The sharing of resources is one of the most exciting possibilities for general practice. It could lead to a uniformity of (high) standards, one of the chief aims of PCGs. It would fit well into the concept of joint training across the PCG and of organisational development. However, there is also the potential problem of divided loyalties and who would have first call on a shared resource in case of difficulty (e.g. through sickness).

PCGs at levels 1 and 2 will be developing longer-term plans and service agreements with providers, but all this via the health authority. For those that decide to proceed to level 3 by becoming free-standing bodies and to level 4 by taking on the additional responsibility for the provision of community services, there will be more autonomy. Primary care will inevitably have to change to move forward. What is important is how primary care practitioners adapt to these changes.

Primary care trusts

As PCGs develop into primary care trusts, there will be less of a role for health authorities – we are already seeing the implications for this in the proposed sharing of certain administration functions across health authority boundaries. Models of shared administration could be shared across practice boundaries. It is possible to envisage a setting in the future where primary care is delivered from multiple sites, but is administered centrally.

Independent contractor status

The implications are obvious – the independent contractor status is theoretically subsumed into the PCG. This would appeal to some doctors, but would probably be resisted by the majority. However, if GPs want to remain at the centre of the changes, then by being involved they have the opportunity to shape those changes. The Government has agreed to the central role doctors and nurses have to play in these reforms. They are aware that planning can be carried out most effectively by practitioners with day-to-day contact with patients. The independent contractor status, cherished since 1948, is under threat, but by being involved in the developments it is possible to strengthen rather than weaken this status in the new NHS.

Organisations

The threat to the process is lack of involvement. Developing an organisational structure the size of a PCG is a new experience for primary care. Trusts, social services and businesses in the wider world are used to the idea of organisations of this size, corporate responsibility and shared ownership. PCG success will depend ultimately upon the involvement of all team members. The potential for division must not be forgotten. Territorial behaviour is well-established in the present structures of practice and we will need to be aware of the sensitivity of reallocating resources from one practice to another. The redistribution to meet clearly identified service needs must be managed effectively to avoid the possibility of resentment, non-cooperation and lack of progress on advancement.

Working together, for example prescribing

Prescribing costs in primary care approximate to half the total primary care budget. PCGs are expected to manage their own prescribing budgets and integrate these into the total spending plans of their PCG. The document *GP Prescribing Support*,[1] a resource document and guide for the new NHS, has been published to enable PCGs to look at their prescribing habits and activities with a view to utilising cost-effective models to maximise cash limited funds available for drug costs.

So, what does it mean to PCGs? One of the underlying themes is the enhanced role of the community pharmacist, the corporate responsibility of the PCG and the role that the National Institute of Clinical Excellence (NICE), via the Commission for Health Improvement (CHIMP) will have to play in monitoring this area.

Rational prescribing

GPs spend significant resources on the prescriptions they issue. The opportunity therefore arises to look carefully at prescribing habits to make maximum use of the scarce resources available (at present, £4 500 000 of the £9 000 000 budget for primary care is spent on prescribing costs). The explosion of medication and treatments available to GPs has mushroomed in the last four years. Until now, the responsibility for managing and informing prescribing advice has rested with the individual practitioner and practice, with limited collaboration from the health authority, pharmaceutical and medical advisors.

Both fundholding and non-fundholding practices have had an incentive to make savings. The former have been more successful in containing drug costs with a direct link between savings made and money available to the practice. Non-fundholders were less successful in containing costs with only a proportion of their savings being available for the practice.

Prescribing support

PCGs can use prescribing support to enable them to make best use of the prescribing budget element of the unified budget. By building on the work of the practices and hospitals that have already developed formularies, it can be envisaged that all PCGs will be able to meet their population prescribing needs while remaining within a cash limited unified budget.

Benefits

What are the benefits to the busy GP in following this path? In all likelihood it will be more and more difficult to have individual personal formularies – the BNF will become a source reference for information rather than the 'personal' formulary. With the development of PCG formularies comes hard work. It will, however, lead to potential gains for patients by:

- using the best medicine available
- individual tailoring of treatment plans
- evidence-based prescribing and therapy
- avoiding unnecessary prescribing and hence iatrogenic illness.

And for GPs through:

- utilising the skills of the pharmacist
- the chance to spend more time on the consideration of patients' needs
- a reduction in inappropriate demand.

Clinical governance

All GPs will be required to meet certain minimum standards. Prescribing will be a key area where targets will be set. Prescribing support will help the busy doctor prescribe appropriately, effectively and to the correct population.

Closer working

Developing PCG formularies will be an educational exercise. As well as a rational prescribing exercise practice teams will be able to discuss 'best options' for specific conditions. Vital to these discussions is the ability to allow for change, individualism and variations. The process of deciding the formulary will, in itself, be a teambuilding exercise.

Resolving primary and secondary care issues

Until now a significant percentage of prescribing in primary care has been instigated by the hospital practitioner. With the unification of primary and secondary budgets it could be envisaged that cost-effective and seamless patient care will be possible. Any prescribing policy will need to cross the interface between primary and secondary care. At present, the primary care formulary is larger than the secondary care formulary. However, a formulary in secondary care will need to be consistent with that in primary care. There will need to be specific agreements on branded drugs offered by pharmaceutical companies to trust pharmacies as loss leaders. There will need to be adherence to policies set up by groups such as joint formulary groups, the monitoring of which could be done by the hospital pharmacist working with the PCG lead pharmacist.

Continuing medical education

It is important that there is an educational element in the methodology adopted for looking at prescribing activity. This not only enhances the activity but also allows the PCG stakeholders to demonstrate the elements of clinical governance have been taken into consideration.

Community pharmacist

The key player in prescribing support is the (community) pharmacist. It is envisaged that he or she will offer increasing advice to both patients and PCGs on their prescribing, reviewing medication on a regular basis especially for those with repeat prescriptions.

For example:

- **Brown bag review** – the patients bring all the medication they have to the surgery or, if not able to attend, are visited at home. Seventy five percent of all prescriptions are issued as repeats. Inevitably, pharmacists find many unused and unnecessary medications. It is likely that PCGs will be particularly interested in this area.
- **Review of recent hospital discharge patients by pharmacists** – this would ensure that patients are taking their medication correctly, not getting confused and that any discrepancies between prescribed medication from the hospital, GP and non-prescription medication are addressed. Any drug interactions can also be identified. It is important that patients do not restart medication taken before admission but not included in their discharge treatment until the correct regime has been decided.
- **Nursing and residential home review** – these institutions frequently display the problems of poly-pharmacy. GPs are often aware of the difficulties but they are not always easy to resolve. For PCGs where there are large numbers of nursing and residential homes, the implications for extra work are enormous. If PCGs have formularies, any review will need to take this into account and decide the pace of change towards an agreed goal.

Prescribing and cost (PACT) data

Pharmacists could work alongside practitioners using the data on their prescribing habits to audit specific areas. This would be one of the most important means of monitoring whether practices are working towards the formulary and guidelines agreed. Further, it would be a means of assessing cost-effectiveness.

In-house clinics

In-house pharmacist and nurse-run clinics to review medication and prescribing might be developed to allow GPs to provide longer patient consultations where appropriate. This would allow a more holistic approach to their treatment plans. The ultimate aim would be to look at ways of improving health by lifestyle changes, alternative methods of improving illness and preventing illness without recourse to drug therapy.

Other routes towards prescribing reduction

Alternative (non-drug) treatments may be tried, although careful consideration as to cost effectiveness should be taken.

- **Stress management** training may be identified as a means of need reduction (e.g. the need for antidepressants, anxiolytics and antihypertensives).
- **Exercise programmes** leading to a reduction in weight, blood pressure, strokes and cardiovascular disease.
- **Health inequalities.** It should be recognised that healthcare is not always the major determinant of health. By reducing health inequalities in other areas (e.g. fortification of flour with folic acid, reduction in traffic) the government or local authorities may have an effect on prescribing.

Important areas to support prescribing

- **Proper resourcing** of information on drug treatments. The PCG should ensure that there is proper distribution of the correct guidelines (e.g. *Drug and Therapeutics Bulletin*, Merec, local prescribing information) or may wish to ask a community pharmacist to condense these into key points for the busy GP and pharmacist.
- **Guidelines and protocols** might be one of the more far-reaching changes suggested to the way we practice. Joint working between community pharmacists and general practice on developing practice guidelines for treatment of certain conditions, repeat prescribing review and the treatment of minor ailments could be based upon guidelines from NICE.
- **Repeat prescribing** – 75% of all prescriptions are issued as repeats. It is inevitable, therefore, that PCGs will look to this area with special interest. Cost savings here are potentially the largest. To ensure that this is dealt with most effectively, community pharmacists and GPs are advised to look at monitoring and reviewing prescriptions on a regular basis.
- **Prescriptions by computer** – the resource suggests that each practice's computer is adapted to a formula, which may reflect the PCG formula. This will be possible to

delegate to a pharmacist, but a word of caution needs to be exercised here: the prescriber who signs the prescription is responsible (in law) for the script. Use of the Prodigy system for prescribing support may augment this.

Developing prescribing in practices

PCGs will need to have effective representation – probably either a GP or pharmacist – on local committees (e.g. drugs and therapeutic committees (DTC) and area prescribing committees (APC)) that look at prescribing. It will be important when developing the local formulary and looking at individual GP prescribing that this is dealt with in a supportive way. GPs may not respond positively to being told they are not matching their peers. It is vital that their prescribing, like their referral patterns, are looked at sensitively, objectively and as part of an overall picture of their medical practice. Support should be constructive and positive rather than critical and negative. Development of prescribing support is likely to be at PCG not individual level. To start with it will be advisable to review practices that have already utilised prescribing support. This will enable the PCG to draw on the positive aspects and tackle those areas where an early 'win' is possible. To make these changes work, all participants must be involved, feel they are involved and want to be involved. There will be no new money to fund this, the money will come from:

- prescribing budgets
- other elements of PCG allocations (e.g. management allowance)
- GMS monies
- other health authority funding streams
- exchange of services, e.g. use a trust pharmacist and in return do extra work for the trust
- practice development funds.

Conclusion

Once the PCG has agreed on the service it needs, it will have to find a suitable professional to lead this role. It may need to recruit a pharmacist or, better still, use a local community pharmacist. This person should be delegated as the PCG prescribing lead. He or she will need to be introduced to individual practices and ensure that the members of the practice team are all aware of the role of the prescribing supporter. There will need to be joint ownership of the activities, a shared agreement to participate and implement any change suggested. Care must be taken to ensure that where authority is delegated, e.g. to 'alter medication on behalf of the doctors', that all participants are happy.

As this is a major change in primary care it will need to be developed sensitively. Do not be too ambitious at first. If a PCG is predicting an overspend, look for quick fixes first. All this has to be monitored, the PCG will be responsible for ensuring due probity and accountability.

Do not plan rapid change. The pace will depend on the diversity of the practices within your PCG, the commitment of the various players and the available resources to make this occur. Plan for achievable gains and do not ignore areas considered as losers. Finally, bring all variables together to try and maximise your potential.

Primary care investment plan

Guidance has outlined the need for PCGs to develop, by January 2000, a primary care investment plan (PCIP). This will need to take into consideration the aims and aspirations of the health authority (through the HImP), the PCG itself (through its own aims and objectives) and each individual practice. The clinical governance programme for the next year will describe the priorities for quality improvement. This will have to link in with the PCIP which will have to:

- describe how spending in GMS will be used and can be protected
- act as a planning document for primary care development
- demonstrate how the investment programme will increase equity and quality
- show how (cost-effective) practice-based services are to he handled in the coming year with the emphasis being on widening provision, e.g. in-house physiotherapy.

The PCIP is clearly going to have to include all practices in its development. This will need considerable communication and co-ordination skills by its main authors (likely to be the PCG chief executive and chair of the board). Where disagreements arise there will need to be a means of making a final decision. PCGs may like to agree upon the principles of the PCIP *before* they look at any effects they have on individual practices. This should avoid bias or lobbying.

What should be in the primary care investment programme?

- **Overview/introduction**   This should give a clear idea on the priorities for the forthcoming year.
- **Premises**   This section should have a description of the current position, existing problems and the main plans for development this year. Some comparative data between practices may be useful to move towards some equity, e.g. number of consulting rooms per doctor or per 1000 patients, the presence or absence of a meeting room, the state of repair of premises. It would be reasonable to look at what the priorities for subsequent years are.
- **Staff**   A description of the current position, current problems and the main plans for the forthcoming year. Comparative data may be easier when looking at staff numbers and costs against formulae (presumably inherited from the health authority). However, whether the formulae are agreed by all practices and how movement towards target is to be achieved are two contentious areas that will need careful negotiation.

- **IM&T**   It is highly likely that non-fundholding practices have had the smallest investment in new IM&T in previous years. Therefore, they will hope to get first claim on any IM&T development money. However, since the pace of change in IT equipment is so rapid, and all practices will need NHS net access in the future, all practices will require some IT investment. Clearly, this section should reflect the National IM&T strategy.
- **Secondary care services and out of hours**   Any development of 'secondary care' services need to be included here. Some financing of this will come from Section 36 funding. The development of out of hours provision and an equalisation of access across the PCG should be discussed, e.g. nurse triage.
- **Savings**   A strategy on how savings will be spent. This should reflect the savings the PCG will receive and those held by practices. Although the latter will be for the practice to use as they wish, it would certainly be important if the use of savings is co-ordinated.
- **Quality initiatives**   How the PCG will improve quality in the forthcoming year, e.g. those topics highlighted within the clinical governance agenda. This will probably include prescribing and so a description of this strategy will be needed.

Primary care – the future

Working with social services

It has long been realised, but only recently stated by government, that there is a link between health and social welfare. In 1997, the Government recognised this link officially with the appointment of a Public Health Minister to co-ordinate services across Whitehall. And the Government is also committed to exploring the possibilities of merging health and social service budgets. It is well recognised in housing that a long tradition of involving tenants in discussions can help inform users' views in the decision-making process.

To extrapolate this into PCGs implies that a community-based approach can extend users' influence and lead to the development of practical services. The PCG Board has a local authority representative who is there to bring the views, experience and planning natural to social service departments. There is a move towards the development of more streamlined and smaller social service boundaries. It is no coincidence that there is an alignment between many PCG boundaries and those of social services. Cross-boundary issues would need to be resolved for a complete devolvement of budgets and planning down to this level but the scene has been set. Further, the role of county council input into social service budget levels may be of some concern. Many areas have seen a drastic cut in social service budgets to ensure education budgets are unharmed. This cut would certainly affect the health budget with an increase in those waiting for nursing home care and an inability to care for those at home without adequate care packages.

Initially though, PCGs will work alongside social services. They will have involvement in the local planning agendas of social service departments and will develop reciprocal arrangements on PCGs. Developing and delivering a range of core packages across the health/social service boundaries will be used to point PCGs and social services towards unified budgets. Examples of this are becoming more popular, such as healthy walking as an adjunct to cardiac rehabilitation, weight reduction programmes, stroke recovery, etc. The theme is that there are more diverse ways to improve the nation's health than by the conventional primary/secondary care interface methods.

Housing is another area where health can be improved without recourse to medicine. The reduction in tuberculosis this century is probably due to improved housing conditions. An improvement in housing conditions for those with conditions affected by a poor environment (e.g. osteoarthritis, obstructive airways disease) may have more effect than medical input. PCGs will need to consider such issues at length and in some depth.

Primary care development – future options

So far in this chapter the impact of PCGs on primary care development has been viewed with the assumption that the primary care team will remain unaltered, with no change in its focus, make-up or the individual roles each member plays.

Within the framework of the White Paper[2] it is possible to envisage different organisational arrangements to facilitate the delivery of primary care. Primary Care Act Pilot Schemes, a new group of which are about to start, were set up to evaluate different working arrangements within primary care. Delphi surveys carried out by the Workforce Planning Project at the Public Health Resource Unit in Oxford, with a Delphi consultation exercise between the Thames Valley Faculty and LMC Chairman of the Oxford Deanery, have looked at the impact of PCGs on primary care development. Perhaps more importantly they have also considered the possible scenarios over the next 5–10 years. It is important when planning a workforce to take into consideration the possible workforce make-up in 5–10 years as much as the possible roles that would be available.

Primary care team

The starting point is the primary care team with the GP as the self-employed independent contractor who acts as leader and a central hub to the team. In the team there are employed practice nurses, a practice manager, secretaries and receptionists (and a dispenser in the case of a dispensing practice). Larger practices may have other employees, such as computer support staff or a fund manager. Attached to the practice are the district nurses, midwives and health visitor team. With PCGs, the primary healthcare team will be part of a larger organisation, working together, collaborating and co-operating. This may seem to be a tall mountain to climb – practices have traditionally been competitive, concerned that patients would move from one GP to another, now they will be working together for their patient's welfare.

The role of the GP in the future may change with the expansion of nurse practitioners. Further, the new primary care physician could be employed as a salaried clinician. They may have an equal say in the running of the team rather than a more controlling influence. Indeed, they may find themselves being managed in a way previously unknown to GPs.

With PCGs (or trusts) there will be a role for the financial stakeholder, as is the current position, but they may be fewer in number with the PCG/T employing a number of salaried doctors who may work at more than one practice. Recent surveys, including that of *The Lost Doctors* carried out by the Public Health Resource Unit in Oxford, have shown there are many doctors who are trained as GPs but who do not want to be principals at the moment.[3] National figures suggest there are around 7000 non-principals. Some doctors will want their commitment to be part time, this is likely to rise when 70–80% of newly qualified GPs are women. They, along with their colleagues, are voicing considerable concerns about their status in the practice with respect to their full-time colleagues. To enable these changes to occur, there must be a culture change in both the expectations of the public and the expectations of the profession. Certain core values will need to be encouraged whatever the role of the GP. For instance, the need to have developed a robust programme of continuing professional development will help meet the terms of clinical governance. Most importantly, the relationship between patient and doctor should be preserved in some form. Although it may not be exactly the same, GPs must not forget their role as 'the generalist', their expertise in consulting and their position as the family doctor.

The various roles in the primary care team will be re-evaluated over the next year or two. It must be remembered though that in most cases the first contact with the NHS will continue to be via primary care. But from this point the patient will have access to a highly trained multidisciplinary health and social care team. The team will not only deal with the healthcare needs of the individual, but will be evaluating the healthcare needs of the PCG populations, ensuring that the messages of health promotion and disease prevention are transmitted and understood by the population they serve.

As primary care changes it is quite possible that patient access to the team will change. The first consultation is less with the GP, who then refers on to their primary care colleague, and increasingly with the actual person best suited to treat their problem. To enable this improved service, team members will have to be able to value the individual contributions of each member. The new models of delivering primary care seen in the Primary Care Act pilots will need to be evaluated and developed.

Primary care development will rely on the development of skills across a wider number of team members. Skills shortages will be an impediment to change. New roles will evolve for team members not currently involved in these areas. To facilitate this there will need to be more shared learning and training across the disciplines.

The effect of PCGs on primary care development will be widespread. One of the most important areas where PCGs can have a beneficial effect is on recruitment and retention.

Robust, well-structured career opportunities with personal development plans will be a strong motivator. Flexibility in employment patterns will attract people into primary care. This will be achievable by the PCG, its resource allocation to staff and premises being able to develop the team. A wise PCG will look to the evidence via library and database searches to see if their individual ideas have been piloted before. The evaluation of such pilots will be invaluable when assessing the development needs of their own particular PCG.

Ten years' time

How will potential patients access primary care and what will be the outcome of their access?

The patient will access the computerised appointment system via their digital television combined Internet link. They will choose from a menu of providers that the system informs them are appropriate to their needs. Today they are offered appointments with the occupational therapist, dietician, pharmacists or social worker. All these have skills particular to their problem. The patient can then make the appointment himself or herself or, if they feel the need for further assistance, ask the online receptionist to help them.

It is possible that today's problem could be dealt with online using the online decision-making process. The software will have answered their question. It is likely that a hybrid of primary and secondary care activities will be available for the patient with specialisation in different practices. With the technology available today a virtual clinic is possible without the expensive relocation of team players on to one site. This would utilise the advances brought with the NHSnet, telemedicine and other computerised access software, all of which will be voice-activated.

It is only just over 30 years ago that GPs had no team except a district nurse and midwife attached to the practice. All other services were accessed via secondary care; appointments and information were part of a futuristic vision that has now become everyday practice.

Conclusion

Hopefully, this chapter has given you some insight into the effects PCGs can have on primary care development. *The New NHS: modern, dependable*[2] and the paper *Our Healthier Nation*[4] have ushered in potentially the biggest changes in the methods of healthcare provision since the birth of the NHS in 1948.

The ability to build on and develop the best in primary care, to work together and co-operate offers great opportunities. To realise these it is incumbent upon all the players in

PCGs to respect their colleagues, listen to their fears and aspirations and to build on their strengths in a non-threatening, non-confrontational way to provide excellent, first class healthcare to the public.

The development of PCGs could be seen as a threat to GPs. With any threat there are also opportunities. There is a chance to develop the role of community-based GPs with an expansion of their skills, taking on many areas currently the preserve of the hospital doctor. Further, they can share the responsibility and care of hitherto GP activities and responsibilities with other members of the primary healthcare team.

The changes in the working conditions for GPs and their colleagues are perhaps the most threatening. By keeping informed and involved they should be able to shape any change to suit their needs.

References

1 NHS Executive (1998) *GP Prescribing Support*. NHSE, Leeds.

2 Secretary of State for Health (1997) *The New NHS: modern, dependable*. Stationery Office, London.

3 Anglian/Oxford NHSE (1998) *The Lost Doctors: a study of doctors not working as principals in general practice*. PHRU, Oxford.

4 Department of Health (1998) *Our Healthier Nation*. Stationery Office, London.

CHAPTER NINE

Health needs assessment and Health Improvement Programmes

Paul Johnstone

Introduction

This chapter looks at what a health needs assessment is, why primary care groups (PCGs) should assess the needs of their population, how to plan and implement a needs assessment using a clear and simple approach, and how this can underpin Health Improvement Plans (HImPs).

This assumes that your PCG is planning a needs assessment with a number of other partners, including

- the local health authority and public health department
- hospitals
- the local authority
- other professionals from other sectors
- users and the general public.

The chapter covers the basics and provides a signpost to more detailed explanation, if required. Above all, time and resources are needed to achieve useful health needs assessments.

Why assess needs?

Most doctors and nurses have been trained to care for individual patients. Through professional training and clinical experience, we have developed a systematic approach to assessing symptoms, making diagnoses, assessing needs and planning care. Although less developed, a similar approach is applied to populations or larger groups. Health needs assessment is a systematic approach to assessing needs in populations using a number of methods, ranging from consulting the general public to technical epidemiological approaches. By prioritising areas for development and planning how specific services can change, a needs assessment will aim to improve health and healthcare in the local population.

A brief history of needs assessment

The desire that the NHS should be a needs-led service started at its inception in 1948. There have been a number of attempts to reduce the inequalities of funding, for example the Resource Allocation Working Party formula (RAWP). However, the science of 'needology' was the preserve of sociologists, public health academics and economists and has rarely been put into routine practice. When the purchaser–provider split was introduced, purchasing decisions based on the needs of populations to achieve 'health gain' came into focus. Public health practitioners, with their training and origins in epidemiology, disease control and health promotion, developed a number of techniques to assess population needs. The 1990 NHS Act required health authorities 'to assess needs of their population and to use these to set priorities and improve health'. At the same time, there is greater interest in involving the general public in shaping services, and a number of techniques have been developed to assess health needs from the user's perspective.[1]

Needs assessments in primary care

Health needs assessments have rarely been developed in primary care. However, the powerful combination of primary care knowledge and the public health approach to assessing needs has been recognised. In the early days, GPs such as Julian Tudor-Hart and John Fry pioneered needs assessments in primary care.

The GP fundholding initiative subsequently put primary care at the front end of the NHS. However, many of these practices emphasised efficient purchasing of services, rather than needs assessments and developing services around health needs. The advent of PCGs presents another opportunity to build on these experiences. One aspect of the

Government's new policy is that access to services should be based on 'need and need alone'; one feature of PCGs will be to plan, commission and monitor local health services to meet local needs.[2]

The basics

Needs assessment – a definition

There are a number of definitions but, in essence, a needs assessment is the following. A method that:

- is objective, valid and a systematic approach
- involves a number of professionals and the general public
- involves using different sources and methods of collecting and analysing information (ranging from epidemiological, qualitative and comparative methods)

which aims to:

- describe health problems in a population and differences within and between different groups
- learn more about the needs and priorities of the local population
- identify unmet need
- identify inequalities in health and access to services
- determine priorities for action
- identify services where people are able to benefit from healthcare or from wider social and environmental change
- make changes to meet unmet needs
- tailor health services resources used in the most efficient way to benefit and improve the health of the population (clinical and cost-effectiveness)
- incorporates users' and the general public's perspectives
- balance clinical, ethical and economic considerations, i.e. what should be done, what can be done and what can be afforded
- influence policy, inter-agency collaboration or research and development priorities.

Why is it important?

With time, the NHS and health systems across the world face similar pressures. These are:

- the rising cost of healthcare
- recent medical advances which show demonstrable benefit
- people are getting older and need more care
- rising expectations.

At some time, most countries, even those with market economies, such as the USA, face similar dilemmas. These are:

- available resources are limited
- people have inequitable access to healthcare
- inverse care law, i.e. people whose needs are greatest are least likely to have access to care (and vice versa)
- concern about appropriateness, effectiveness and quality.

The challenge for PCGs, which in many respects are taking on the mantle of health authority and public health for populations, is to make decisions that maximise the benefit for the resources available to all its population. Needs assessment helps this decision making. We describe three stages to this approach.

Three steps to assessing needs

- Step 1: define the population and its boundaries and look at routine data from different sources to start the ball rolling.
- Step 2: involve the general public and users, and from this prioritise a hit list to analyse.
- Step 3: look at specific areas of care in more detail using epidemiology, with recommendations for changes and how this should be financed.

Later in the chapter we will look at each of these stages in more detail. But before that we need to consider some things which a needs assessment is not:

- a technical preserve of health authorities and public health departments (technical skills are often exaggerated and all that is required is basic numeracy, common sense, time and some resources), or
- a distraction for putting off difficult decisions.

Need for health versus need for healthcare

The World Health Organisation (WHO) definition of health is wide; it is not just the absence of disease, but physical, mental and social well being. Clearly most of us would be of ill health on a rainy Monday morning in winter. Our health is determined by many factors outside the health service. Individual needs for health include the needs for a job, to live in a house, to pay for food and health education to avoid damaging behaviour such as smoking.

Our influence on these may appear well outside the immediate control of those of us working in health services. However, if doctors and nurses in PCGs see, and have an understanding of, the consequences of these factors, they can help to tackle wider problems. For this reason the WHO Alma Ata Declaration[3] stated that one way to achieve the

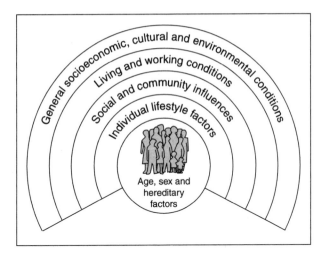

Figure 9.1: The wider determinants of health and their relationship to individuals.

goal of health for all (by the year 2000) was through working with other sectors, such as education, social services, planning and housing, and the voluntary sector. This is one of the reasons why the NHS White Paper[2] states that HImPs should be developed with other partners from other sectors.

Theory versus pragmatism in needs assessment

There are a number of theories about needs and needs assessment. It may be useful to have a wider understanding of these theories but it is not essential for carrying out a needs assessment.

There are broadly three views of need:

- The *economist's view* – need is traded off with desire to pay someone to do something about the need; needs are always greater than resources.
- The *sociologist's view* – need is either felt or perceived and behaviour leads to meeting this need.
- The *public health view* – using epidemiology and statistics to quantify numbers of affected people, and the services available. This view is described as identifying the *population's ability to benefit* from medical or social interventions and how these services can improve health.

While all three give insights into how to measure need and what to expect from a needs assessment, the public health view of need has been the most highly developed to become a practical tool for needs assessments. Before looking at this, we consider what happens to some people in their daily endeavours to seek healthcare services.

Need demand and supply

It is important to distinguish between need (i.e. what people can benefit from to improve their health) and demand (i.e. what people ask for, are willing to pay for or might wish to use in a system of free care), and from supply (i.e. what is actually provided). This helps to classify health service interventions into whether they are needed, demanded or supplied (or a combination). Most information we have from health service data is on supply (i.e. utilisation rates) or demand (e.g. patient satisfaction surveys), rather than on need. It is important, as healthcare commissioners, to bring together needs, supply and demand, in other words, what people ask for, they will benefit from and can be supplied (*see* Figure 9.2).

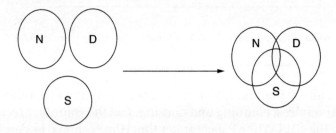

Figure 9.2:   The relation between needs, supply and demand.

Public health view of need

This approach is concerned with assessing 'the population's ability to benefit from health care.'[4–6] 'Ability to benefit' is important, because as commissioners of healthcare it is crucial that there is some benefit (either immediate or in the future; physical, psychological, personal or communal). This benefit is measured as strength of evidence of effectiveness and cost-effectiveness. It should be remembered that for some interventions, the benefits are difficult to measure, although there is research to show their effectiveness (*see* Box 9.1). Quality of caring (e.g. sympathy) may make a patient feel better but is not easily measured. As this is the cornerstone of primary care it should not be forgotten but put into context. An 'intervention' can range from health promotion to diagnosis, palliation or treatment. It is argued that assessing needs is only useful when there is an intervention that can provide benefit.

Later in the chapter we will consider epidemiological needs assessment in more detail. However, we will first look at planning a needs assessment, the value of routine data and involving the public.

> **Box 9.1:** Measuring benefit
>
> Benefit can be measured and described in terms of outcomes to patients. This is scientifically determined through controlled trials, such as randomised control trials, which avoid the risk of bias. Measuring benefit can be technically difficult in a population. Imagine two individuals, one a 79-year-old woman and the other a 40-year-old woman, both with arthritis of the hip. Both would benefit from a hip operation but the 40-year-old would probably benefit more than the 79-year-old (although the costs to the NHS may be the same). Cost in terms of risk of operation complications and increased morbidity would be higher for the older person who may not want such an operation. Benefit is also difficult because it changes with time. For example, someone with complete sensory neural deafness ten years ago would have a need for social care and education but not for medical care, since there was no intervention they could benefit from. Now, of course, we have the cochlea-implant programme, and the patient can now benefit from medical care.

Planning a needs assessment

How do we go about assessing need? What makes a successful needs assessment? This section moves from the theories of need to a practical approach. Reconsider the three basic steps to a needs assessment by having a go at the exercise in Box 9.2.

> **Box 9.2:** Exercise
>
> Imagine you are standing on the edge of a refugee camp in Africa. The camp houses 100 000 people. There is overcrowding and illness. As a doctor or nurse, how would you best spend your time to help the refugees?
>
> Answer: start by collecting some basic information (what are the boundaries of the camp, death rates and causes of death?). Talk to people, leaders, aid workers and patients, to get a feel for their needs. Then look at specific programmes to meet these needs, for example programmes for immunisation, tuberculosis, oral rehydration. Finally, ask what services already exist for the refugees. Is this meeting need? Can it be improved to do so? Think how this approach could be used in your PCG.
>
> *Suggested outline for answers*
>
> 1 Global approach
>   - define the population
>   - identify any easily available information
> 2 Then involve users and the public
>   - overview of health and social needs
>   - prioritise
> 3 Finally, focus on priority in more detail using epidemiology

We have identified three practical steps:

- Step 1. Think about the big picture:
  - define the population
  - identify any easily available information.
- Step 2. Involve users and the public:
  - overview of health and social needs
  - prioritise.
- Step 3. Focus on priority, which could be:
  - a speciality, e.g. mental health
  - a disease
  - a client group
  - groups waiting for interventions (e.g. hip operations)
  - vulnerable groups (ethnic minorities)
  - socially deprived addressed by inequity.

Each of these is considered below. But before that, think through what actually makes a needs assessment successful (Box 9.3).

Box 9.3:   Exercise: write down what you think would make a needs assessment successful

The following list may help:

- start simple then build up
- need time, resources and commitment
- involve other agencies (hospitals, voluntary sector, health authority, media)
- audit and education
- integrate into planning cycle to coincide with important management decisions
- successful action following the assessment

Planning a needs assessment

Therefore a checklist for planning should include:

- define aim
- identify community
- identify resources, including personnel
- any training required?
- plan method
- routine data
- how are we going to involve other agencies and the public?
- prioritise
- focused topics
- additional surveys

- analyse and report
- action plan (or a HImP).

In summary, planning a needs assessment is about planning a process and philosophy of working, which may be different from the way we have worked before in primary care. It is about working and respecting the views of others, including agencies and patients (or the general public), and about being systematic, looking at big picture problems and then focusing on priorities.

Step 1: Baseline information

This section considers the first step, finding routine available information and how it can be used.

Three questions should be asked at the start:

1 What are the boundaries of the area for a needs assessment? We need a map and information on demography.
2 What are people dying of or why are they consulting their doctors? We need routine data on deaths, death rates and hospital data on admissions.
3 What else do we need? We need to discuss the findings from questions 1 and 2 above with others in primary care to establish further information required.

A surprising amount of data are already available and will give quite a lot of information to 'start the ball rolling'. Figures 9.3–9.7 show some sources of routinely available

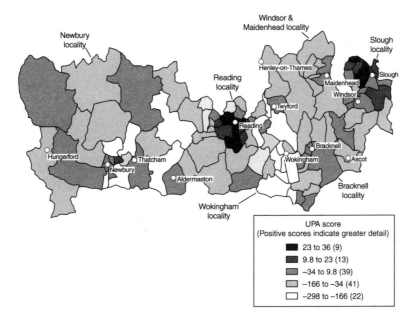

Figure 9.3: UPA score.

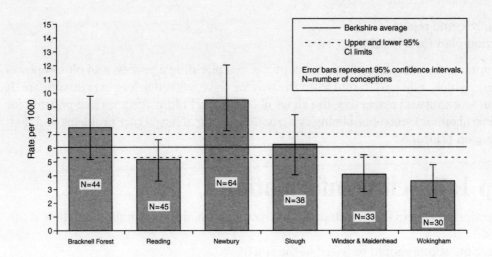

Figure 9.4: Conception rate in girls aged 13–15 per 1000, 1993–95. This graph confirmed suspicions in primary care that teenage pregnancies were high in a small number of wards in Reading and Bracknell.

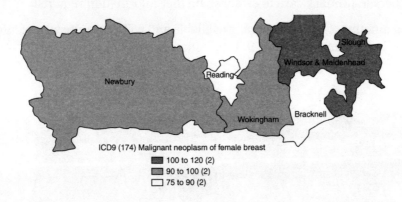

Figure 9.5: Standard mortality ratios (SMRs) by locality. Deprivation and its relationship to ill health were confirmed in this map, showing that deaths from breast cancer were highest in Slough, the most deprived locality in Berkshire.

information, which may be accessed by health authority, hospital library or local authority information departments. Such information can be produced in packs and used in meetings. Discussions about the data can lead to a consensus on what areas are priorities. There will be opportunities to confirm or refute existing knowledge in primary

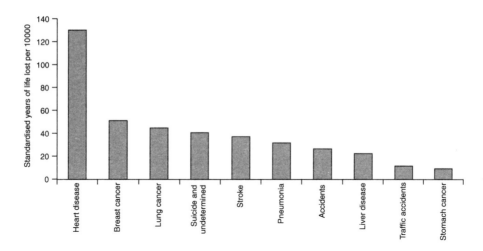

Figure 9.6: Age-standardised average annual years of life lost up to age 75 per 10 000 residents by selected causes of death (deaths registered in Slough 1994–96). It is possible to calculate how many years were lost in a population due to premature deaths. This graph shows ten causes of death that create the greatest volume of years of life lost due to premature death. These demonstrate, for example, that while heart disease and stroke are the most common causes of death, high levels of years of life lost are generated by breast cancer, accidents and suicides. This arises from the fact that these deaths often occur at a relatively early age.

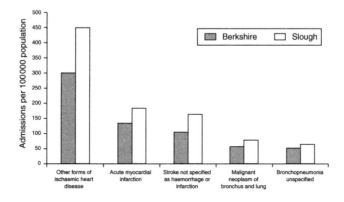

Figure 9.7: Hospital admission rates for Slough residents for the top five causes of death (1997–98). Data on use of services, i.e. demanded and supplied, also give a good idea of need. This graph shows that for the top five causes of death, Slough residents were admitted to hospital at a higher rate than the rest of Berkshire.

care, especially the views of health visitors, district nurses, community mental health teams and social workers. It can also be a starting point to involve the public. Figures 9.3–9.7 show some of the data that were available to inform a needs assessment and HImP in one district.

Advantages and disadvantages to routine information

Such data are readily available and can provide a snapshot of what people die from and why they consult their doctors in a population. They can be used to help bring a wide range of professionals on board with the needs assessment, to start to prioritise topics for action and to begin the process of involving the public.

There are some disadvantages that we should be aware of in our discussions. For example, the data might be quite old (it often takes up to 2 years for routine data to become available), diseases may have been misdiagnosed or not reported, and hospital data may reflect different admission policies for the same condition. Nevertheless it does help to start the process and to approach others who have a contribution.

Step 2: Involving users and the public

Users of health services may have different ideas about what improves their health than health professionals have. This may include having a job, shelter, food or being on a bus route. It is important to acknowledge the limitations to professional knowledge. Through a variety of means this knowledge provides a powerful contribution to a health needs assessment.

Primary care professionals may feel they do not have the time or inclination to do anything about these things and may feel less confident. But if PCGs have the aim of improving health status of these individuals as well as providing services, then at least they need to be identified for action by someone else. Although this stage may seem time-consuming and difficult, involving users and the public can be a rewarding and empowering experience for all involved, which ultimately helps in acting on the findings of a needs assessment.

There are a confusing number of terms for the process, including community appraisals, rapid appraisals and community surveys. Many of the techniques have been pioneered in developing countries and by researchers using so-called qualitative methods, unstructured or semi-structured approaches to understanding behaviours and beliefs and attempting to reduce the biasing effect of measuring health and needs through the eyes of professionals.

Consulting the public is covered in more detail in Chapter 11. However, Boxes 9.4 and 9.5 illustrate some of the approaches that could be used in a needs assessment and some practical steps.

Box 9.4: Getting public involvement

- *Citizens' juries*, selected as representatives of the public or local opinion leaders. Experts give evidence and jurors have an opportunity to ask questions and debate

- *User consultation panels*, local people selected as representatives of the locality. Typical members rotate for a broad range of views. Topics are considered in advance and members are presented with relevant information. Meeting facilitated by a moderator

- *Focus groups*, semi-structured discussion groups of 6–8 people led by a moderator

- *Questionnaire survey*, postal or hand-distributed. Structured questionnaire aims to collect data from a large number of people. Most appropriate when issues behind questions are well known

- *Panels*, large sociologically representative samples (around 100) of a population in a health authority; surveyed at intervals

- *Household surveys*

- *Exit interviews* after a clinic visit, perspective of quality of care or understanding any health messages

- *Interviews* with health workers (people's perceptions of local needs, interviews structured or semi-structured)

Box 9.5: Some practical steps in planning a consultation with the public for a needs assessment

- Summarise existing information from any previous surveys or interviews with the public
- Decide which method will suite the PCG best (*see* Box 9.4)
- Plan the survey with resources, people and time set aside
- Collate information
- Ranking priorities league table
- Meeting to feedback results
- Rank prioritise again

Beware false hopes

The poster in Figure 9.8 comes from a developing country programme, where many needs assessments and surveys had taken place. Alas nothing happened after the surveys.

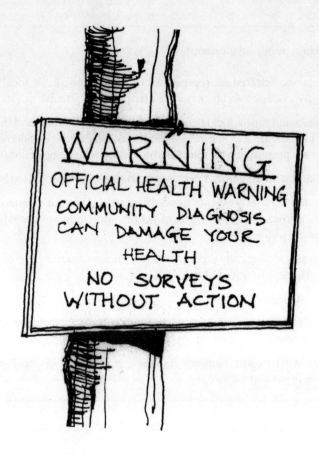

Figure 9.8:   Beware of false hopes.

Prioritising topics

If you have chosen to consult the public, or a smaller groups of professionals, by now you will be getting a clear idea of the top 'hit list' of topics for the PCG. You will also have a larger number of people to help you carry out further detailed work on the topics.

In summary, we may fear some aspects of involving users and the public, particularly the extra burden of work. However, in most cases the dividends are very rewarding. Their involvement will help to provide a wider and more sensitive view of needs in communities and will help the different agencies to develop a common vision for the community.

Step 3: Epidemiological needs assessment

This stage of the needs assessment focuses on specific priorities for the PCG moving from the big to the detailed picture. These priorities may be:

- a speciality, e.g. mental health
- a disease
- a client group
- groups waiting for interventions (e.g. hip operations)
- vulnerable groups (ethnic minorities)
- socially deprived addressed by inequity.

Questions to ask

- What is the problem, size, nature?
- What needs do current services meet?
- Is this what patients want?
- What are the most appropriate, effective solutions?
- What are the resource implications?
- What are the outcomes to evaluate change and criteria for audit success?

To start to answer some of these we need to consider some basic epidemiology.

What is epidemiology and how can it help?

Last[7] defined epidemiology as the study of distribution and determinants of health-related states or events in specific populations and the application of this study to control of health problems. It follows the medical model of health need, viewing need in terms of specific diseases.

In needs assessments we use 'descriptive epidemiology', i.e. where patterns of diseases are described usually in incidence and prevalence. *Incidence* is new cases of disease over a time period (e.g. heart attacks per annum) and *prevalence* is the total number with a condition in the population (i.e. numbers of people with angina per 1000 population).

There are two main types of descriptive surveys:

- *Cross-sectional surveys* or snapshot pictures measure prevalence of current illness conditions or patient views.
- *Longitudinal surveys* measure new cases with time, to assess the incidence of disease, or following-up cases for assessing risk factors over a period of time.

If our descriptions of diseases remain uniform for different areas and at different times, then we need a uniform definition of a 'case'. For most diseases, such as schizophrenia or hypertension for example, there exists a range of severity, from normal to borderline to severe. We have to be clear that the criteria used to define a case in one area are the same as in others areas. For most conditions, there are internationally accepted criteria (e.g. schizophrenia, hypertension, diabetes). For routine data, such as national data described in step 1, criteria for cases have to be consistent to be useful. PCGs should always check that this is true, particularly for data collected in a local survey (e.g. practice computer systems, *see* Chapter 6).

Box 9.6:   Planning an epidemiological survey for a needs assessment

The type of needs assessment survey described above needs a little extra planning. Here is a check list for such a plan:

1   Resources – time and money, plan, staff
2   State aim – what do we want to use this for, what is the disease, what risk factors are being investigated and measured, what is the case definition and which population is of interest?
3   Calculate sample size for survey
4   Choose sample frame and a sample selected (randomly, systematically)
5   Survey instrument should be valid and reliable (repeatable). This can be a question-naire, QOL, physiological measurement or a laboratory test
6   Pilot questionnaire and make adjustments
7   Conduct full survey – ensure high response rate
8   Write up report
9   Disseminate findings

Consider the example in Box 9.7 of a local epidemiological survey in one GP locality commissioning project.

This example demonstrated an epidemiological approach measuring three things:

• The size of the problem: determine how much illness or burden of (in this example, mental) ill health there is in the community by assessing the incidence and prevalence.

• What current services exist to meet this burden? How does provision compare to other areas? Do you think these services meet need or over- or underprovide for the need?

• Are the services effective? If new services are needed to meet unmet need, what works to make a difference?

Box 9.7: An example of a locality prevalence study for a needs assessment of severe mental illness

Aim: to identify needs for specialist care for serious mental illness in one locality, i.e. patients with a diagnosis of schizophrenia, psychosis or severe personality disorder made by a consultant psychiatrist (using DSM criteria)

Method: patients (aged between 15 and 64 years) as cases were identified from GP records. A questionnaire was developed assessing current prevalence, and current levels of care known by GP

Results
- 147 patients with schizophrenia and other psychoses (any type) identified across nine practices (population 43 950)
- prevalence 3.3/1000 (range 1–9/1000)
- 65% were seen by GP in previous 3 months
- 54% were known to have a community psychiatric nurse (CPN) but of these only 40% knew of regular contacts
- 20% had been admitted to hospital in the previous 6 months, of whom one-third were not known to have a CPN

Outcome: the survey led to improved communications between community mental health services and primary care. A review of some recent research by the practices showed that using a 'shared register' of cases for primary and secondary care was beneficial. This was introduced along with liaison CPNs

Questions
1   What sort of epidemiological study was this?
2   What was the definition of case and why was this important?
3   What pitfall should we be aware of in this study?

Answers
1   Prevalence/snapshot
2   Diagnosis by consultant using DSM criteria, important for consistency in a condition which has a wide variation from borderline to severe
3   Variations in case definition, only GP notes used – there may be other cases in the locality not known to GPs

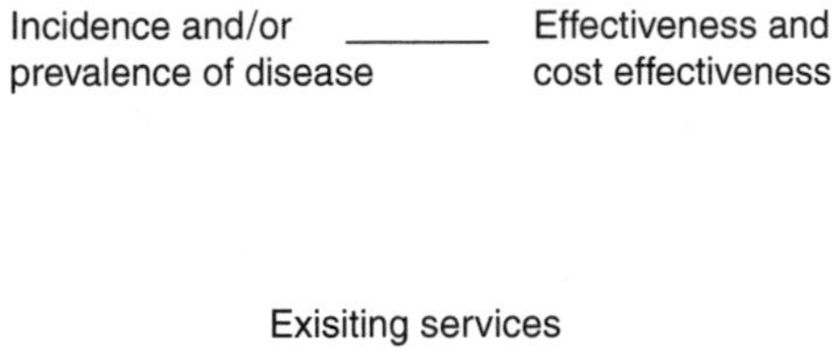

Incidence and/or   _____   Effectiveness and
prevalence of disease   cost effectiveness

Exisiting services

Figure 9.9: The epidemiological approach.

Epidemiological approach in more detail

This approach to measuring needs using epidemiology was refined in the NHS in the early 1990s to support health authorities in their responsibility to 'purchase services according to needs'. Subsequently, a series of practical, off-the-shelf guides to assessing population needs which estimates health, illness and optimal services to meet needs for an average UK population of 250 000 has been published.[8] These guides should be considered and provide a starting point for further investigation and should be used when working with other colleagues, particularly public health colleagues who have had training in this type of needs assessment. The basic steps for an epidemiological based needs assessment are described here.

1   A statement of the problem
    • A disease, client group or risk behaviour for example.
    • Can these be subcategorised, such as primary and secondary prevention of stroke, or mild to severe mental illness, to help focus on the issues?
2   Prevalence and incidence
    • What national data are available? How does the local population compare with others?
    • Are there any local studies to support national data, patient records?
    • Do we have to do a new survey?
    • Can we identify unmet need and overprovision?
3   Services available
    • What services are available for the problem?
    • Try and quantify them. How do these data compare with other similar populations?
4   Models of services
    • Which models of care currently exist?
    • Which other models should be considered?
5   Effectiveness and cost-effectiveness of services
    • Does evidence exist to support models of services (e.g. check Effective Healthcare Bulletins, National Institute of Clinical Effectiveness, the Cochrane Library and other databases).
    • Which model is cost-effective?
6   Recommendations
    • Recommend alternative services which would mean meeting unmet need and reducing oversupply (i.e. health gain for same resources).
    • Influence local policy and relationship between local agencies.

(Adapted from Stevens and Raftery[8])

   Box 9.8 shows an example of an epidemiological-based needs assessment which led to service changes.

Box 9.8:   Developing evidence-based mental health services

Statement of the problem
- A needs assessment was specifically set up to identify the needs of people with serious mental illness and how care could be reprovided following the closure of a large Victorian hospital in the district

Prevalence and incidence
- National data provide local prevalence of serious mental illness (0.3% total population)
- Additional local studies used from trust

Services available
- Services were more dependent on hospitals (for example, lengths of hospital stays were longer than national averages)
- Comparative data suggested under-resourcing and underprovision of community services

Models of services
- Which models of care currently exist? We found a number of community models including community mental health teams, case management
- Which other models should be considered? We wanted to consider assertive care teams, crisis response teams, day care provision and length of hospital stays

Effectiveness and cost-effectiveness of services
- From searches in the Cochrane Library and other databases a multidisciplinary group appraised papers and suggested that assertive care teams were supported with evidence of effectiveness. Case management was found to increase admission rates and not improve mental health

Recommendations
- Assertive care teams and locality-based community mental health teams were recommended with the building of effective community links
- All agencies signed up to the recommendations. An additional £300 000 was provided to develop assertive care teams

---

Identifying overprovision and unmet need

One of the aims of a needs assessment is to find out if there is overprovision of services, and to question whether the money spent on this service could be spent elsewhere, particularly other areas of unmet need. Box 9.9 shows an example of how under- and overprovision of care was identified in general practice in the care of people with secondary heart disease.

As resources for healthcare are always finite, the purpose of this type of needs assessment is to identify health gain, i.e. health improvement can be achieved by reallocating resources as a result of identifying overprovision and unmet need.

Box 9.9:   A survey assessing needs for secondary CHD prevention

Aim: to ensure effective and efficient provision of use of statins in secondary CHD prevention in five practices. According to evidence-based criteria, all patients with a history of heart attacks or angina should receive a statin

Case definition: all patients having had a heart attack or history of angina

Method: all patients with history of heart attacks or angina and those taking statins were identified from practice computers. Their notes were pulled and patients taking statins were recorded and patients with positive histories were recorded

Results: the survey identified a number of patients with positive histories and who were receiving statins appropriately. However, some with CHD were not receiving statins (unmet need) and some who were receiving them did not have a positive history (overprovision)

Outcome: this survey identified patients who would most benefit from an intervention, i.e. who have needs and can benefit from an intervention. It also identified patients who were less likely to benefit, yet were taking statins (oversupply)

Questions
1   How would you plan to ensure that future patients are prescribed statins according to need?
2   Are there other examples of oversupply and unmet need in other areas of healthcare?

Summary

This approach to a health needs assessment is specific to a disease or client group. It aims to systematically identify needs and how services can be optimised to meet these needs using epidemiological information. Such an approach helps to influence policy and management decisions. Success also requires an open mind and a willingness to accept change.

Health improvement: plans and action

How does a needs assessment make a difference? How will it fit into the new NHS developments for HImPs and the day-to-day work of PCGs?

What is a HImP?

The ultimate aim of a HImP is to plan to achieve the aims in *Our Healthier Nation.*[9,10] These are:

- to improve the health of the population as a whole by increasing the length of people's lives and the number of years people spend free from illness
- to improve the health of the worst-off in society and to narrow the health gap.

So far four national priorities have been identified to help meet these aims:

- heart disease and stroke
- accidents
- cancer
- mental health.

Contents of a HImP

These are likely to change with time. Currently, the following information is recommended.

- A description of the small range of local priorities, particularly on health inequalities.
- An agreement with local organisations to act on these priorities.
- A method to show that this action is based on evidence of effectiveness.
- A method to show how progress will be measured.
- A plan for involving the public.
- Describe how it will be used to shape local services.

The first HImPs will be concerned with the first two stages described in this chapter, that is:

- using routine data to assess priorities for the local area
- involving the public and other agencies.

However, how will this influence local policies, change the local service and make a difference?

Son of HImP!

Over the next 3–5 years HImPs will change to tackle three or four specific areas through needs assessment. These are likely to include national priorities mentioned before, namely the National Service Frameworks for coronary heart disease, mental health and cancer, and local priorities if these have not been covered. At this stage epidemiological needs assessments will be needed and will be crucial if HImPs are going to make a difference. Recommendations from more detailed needs assessments will be written into health service financial documents called Service and Financial Frameworks (SaFFs), joint investment plans (these are plans for action by both health authorities and local authorities), social service/local authority plans and the future commissioning plans for PCGs. Having these plans will also allow access to additional money through the proposed NHS Modernisation Fund (*see* Box 9.10).

Box 9.10:   How YOU can influence how NHS money is spent to improve health and health services through needs assessments and HImPs

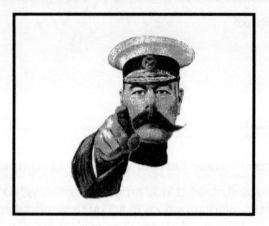

From existing NHS money
Identify overprovision and unmet need through epidemiological needs assessments and redistribute resources. This should be written into the health authority's Service and Financial Frameworks (SaFFs) and future budget plans by PCGs

Combining resources with other agencies
New development planned in social service plans
Joint investment plans (funding of projects by both social services and the NHS)

New money
The NHS Modernisation Fund, which will be released specifically in response to the findings of needs assessments and HImPs

---

The importance of HImPs

There is little doubt that HImPs will be central to the planning over a health authority area. PCGs will have to show that their plans and achievements match those of the HImP. The HImP will prevent PCGs from using all their time to meet their local priorities (although there will be some time for this). However, PCGs will have to learn about fitting in with national and regional priorities which will be reflected within the HImP.

It is unclear how PCG budgets will be established with respect to HImPs. Will monies be top-sliced for HImP priorities or will PCGs have to demonstrate that they are putting suitable amounts of resources into the HImP? For example, the HImP for your health authority has identified the homeless as an important area for PCGs. However, your PCG does not have any homeless within its area. How will this affect your budget? How will this priority be financed?

PCGs must make sure they are able to contribute fully to the HImP. They should ensure that their priorities are included within the HImP. The best way to do this is to provide the evidence that your priorities demonstrate a genuine health need. The best way to do this is through health needs assessment.

Conclusions

A health needs assessment is a systematic process which seeks to identify needs and recommends changes to optimise the delivery of health services. Much can be achieved with a little basic numeracy, common sense and time. It is a process to engage users and the public, and to work with other agencies. This helps to turn simple information into knowledge and to inform how best to commission effective services to make a difference to the health of communities. Above all, it requires an open mind and a willingness to accept change. Assessing needs is described in three steps:

- Step 1: collect and analyse routine data. This tells us what people die from and why they consult their practices, hospitals and social services. This helps to prioritise topics, and allows other partners to get on board and begin to understand needs.
- Step 2: involve a wider participation. Include all practices' staff, social workers, other health workers, and the public and users. Professional views of health needs can differ from the users' views and the involvement of others will allow wider ownership of the process.
- Step 3: focus on one or two priorities, such as a speciality (mental health), a disease (stroke), a client group (teenagers) or a vulnerable, socially deprived group (such as ethnic minorities). Use of epidemiology and local knowledge will answer:
  - How many have the 'disease' (or in client group, etc.) and have health needs which could be met by services and interventions in the community?
  - What services are available at the moment to meet these needs – identify under- and overprovision?
  - What changes are required, based on evidence of effectiveness, to meet these needs? This will help with commissioning decisions about deployment and redeployment of resources.

Each stage plays a central role in the development of the new NHS HImPs and the resources needed or redistributed to improve health and health services.

References

1   National Health Service Executive (1992) *Local Voices: the view of local people in purchasing for health*. Department of Health, London.

2   Secretary of State for Health (1997) *The New NHS: modern, dependable*. Stationery Office, London.

3   World Health Organisation (1975) *The Alma Mater Declaration*. WHO World Health Assembly A28/9. WHO, Geneva.

4   National Health Service Management Executive (1991) *Assessing Health Needs*, (DHA project discussion paper). NHSME, Leeds.

5   Frankel S (1991) The epidemiology of indications. *Journal of Epidemiology and Community Health*. 257–9.

6   Stevens A, Gabbay J (1991) Needs assessment needs assessment. *Health Trends*. **23**: 31–3.

7   Last JM (1988) *A Dictionary of Epidemiology* (2e). Oxford University Press, Oxford.

8   Stevens A and Raftery J (eds) (1994) *Health Care Needs Assessment: the epidemiologically based needs assessment reviews. First series (2 vols)*. Radcliffe Medical Press, Oxford; Stevens A and Raftery J (eds) (1997) *Health Care Needs Assessment: the epidemiologically based needs assessment reviews. Second series (1 vol)*. Radcliffe Medical Press, Oxford.

9   Department of Health (1998) *Our Healthier Nation*. Stationery Office, London.

10   NHS Executive (1998) *Health Improvement Programmes: planning for better health and better health care*. HSC1998/167:LAC(98)23. NHSE, London.

CHAPTER TEN

Working with other agencies

Linda Challis

Primary care groups (PCGs) need to work productively with their partners in local government and the independent sectors. Although some localities are already blessed with excellent collaboration between health and social services, it is still too easy to find examples of suspicion and mistrust underpinned by cumbersome procedures for co-ordination. A witness from the Institute of Health Service Managers quoted by the Health Committee of the House of Commons in its report for 1992–93,[1] claimed that the relationship between GPs and social services staff is:

> ...almost as though they live on different planets, in terms of the language they use and some of the attitudes which are displayed. (Paragraph 124)

Poor linkage between health and social services makes itself felt in every corner of primary care and at the interface between primary and secondary care. The report from the Clinical Standards Advisory Group, *Community Health Care for Elderly People*, published in January 1998,[2] based on 600 interviews about the care received by people with fractured hips, highlighted the problem of cost shunting, the non-implementation of national guidelines on discharge from hospital, and the increased workload on GPs and district nurses which has not been matched by additional funding. The report recommends getting rid of the divide between health and social services, and in particular the illogicality of care provided by social services being means tested and that by the NHS being 'free'. The relevant minister at the time, Paul Boateng, commented that 'the report's recommendations support the thrust of our work to demolish unhelpful barriers between health and social care.'

The flashpoints in the relationship have long been hospital discharge, the use of residential solutions to care problems rather than community-based ones, poor co-ordination resulting in fractured service delivery, and contested claims to budgets as, for

example, in the notorious instance of who should pay for a patient/user to have a bath –
the health service (if so which part of it?) or the social services?

However, it would be an oversimplification to pose the problem as being one of how
doctors get on with social workers.[3] Within social services there is a multiplicity of
occupational groups that have some stake in the provision of social care (e.g. residential
social workers, care managers, day centre managers, home helps, occupational therapists,
counsellors, housing officers, social security staff, and the private and voluntary
sectors), and within the health services there is an even greater array of professional and
occupational groups (e.g. many different kinds of nurses, doctors, midwives, occupational
therapists, physiotherapists, radiotherapists, podiatrists, psychologists, speech therapists,
counsellors and many more).

If the new world of constructive collaboration between PCGs and colleagues in other
parts of the health service, in local government and beyond is to become a reality, then it
might be helpful to learn some of the lessons from past attempts to achieve integrated
planning and care. There is after all a long history of trying to put matters right.

Phase 1 solutions: social service attachments to general practice

Dongray, writing in the *British Medical Journal*,[4] is cited as one of the early examples of
one very popular way of achieving harmonious working together. Her article, published
in 1958, described an attachment to a university medical practice and identified advantages of attachment; namely:

- greater accessibility for the doctors to social services, especially with cases where it
  was not clear to whom a referral should be made, where 'the dominant need is for an
  assessment of the situation on which to base a plan of help' (p 1222)
- the growth of mutual respect and trust
- an excellent place in which to discover unmet need
- carrying out preventive work.

The 1960s and early 1970s saw considerable growth in the number of attachment
schemes (*see* Goldberg and Neill[5]) but by 1979 Marshall and Hargreaves[6] were writing
to warn the unwary of the painful consequences of some attachments. They noted that
'a great many of these projects fail; many cause great anguish to all concerned. This
must be due to inadequate preparation and partly to a failure to recognise the very real
difficulties inherent in these schemes'. There followed a long list of the structural and
professional impediments to collaboration. They also made the useful point that behind
the rhetoric, primary healthcare teams are sometimes not teams at all, that 'the staff are
at loggerheads behind the public facade'.

Beales, writing in a book entitled *Sick Health Centres and How to Make Them Better*,[7]
made similar points and argued that social workers seemed destined to remain outside

the primary healthcare team until '...there is a marked narrowing of the great divide at the administrative heights'. He went so far as to suggest that it was a waste of time and money to allocate space to social services in health centres until such time as reorganisation had occurred. But Beales also noted the importance of personalities in sealing the success or failure of attachments and stressed the importance of attaching only workers who would fit into the health centre.

The themes emerging by the mid-1970s were that further policy effort was needed to create a suitable environment for local schemes to operate effectively. The emphasis switched from local initiative to specific structural change to promote and consolidate co-operation between primary health and social care.

Phase 2 solutions: strategy and structure

More specifically, joint planning and joint finance initiatives at a more strategic level were thought to be what was needed to bring about greater integration. The reorganisation of local government and of the NHS in 1974 provided an opportunity to introduce a new system for collaboration. The machinery consisted of joint consultative committees (JCCs), joint care planning teams and joint finance, with the latter intended to promote community care by reducing the dependence on long-stay hospitals. In the pursuit of a more strategic approach to collaboration, the focus shifted away from attachment schemes to the process of joint planning and joint finance.

There have been a number of studies which have assessed the success of these strategic initiatives.[8-11] The conclusions they reached were very similar, namely that the strategic approach had led to a complex bureaucracy, that the worsening resource base for local government had undermined joint planning, and that there had been both professional and trade union opposition to change.[12]

Nocon[13] studied health and social service authorities' attempts to work together to close a psychiatric hospital. Not only was finance an obstacle to joint work, but so too were the suspicions that each agency had of the other. More specifically, health was fearful that social services was going to cream off resources to fund non-health related activities. While the local authority suspected that the district health authority was acting on behalf of the Conservative Government, trying to transfer responsibilities to local government without an adequate transfer of money to pay for them.

Phase 3 solutions: care management and joint commissioning

The criticisms of joint planning and finance reached a crescendo in the Audit Commission report of 1986[14] and the Griffiths report of 1988.[15] The Audit Commission very firmly pulled the issues of collaboration and joint working back down from the Olympian heights of JCCs to the level of good practice in the primary healthcare team. It saw the existing statutory framework as a barrier to co-operation rather than as an aid to it.

The report, *Making A Reality of Community Care*,[14] argued that the emphasis was on services, not on clients, and that decision making about services was organisationally fragmented and required proposals to be passed up and down substantial hierarchies in both health and social services. In its section on 'Strategic options for consideration' the Commission stated:

> *The objective of any changes should be to create an environment in which locally integrated community care can flourish.*

and that:

> *The management focus should be on local operations rather than (as at present) on the headquarters organisation and joint planning machinery.*

Local initiatives were therefore back in fashion and were underwritten by Sir Roy Griffiths. The pendulum had swung back towards an approach that favoured grass root initiatives. It provided an environment within which ventures like attachments to primary care were no longer seen as tinkering but as a spearhead for the implementation of 'needs-led', rather than 'service-driven', community care.

The experience of the internal market, the development of care planning, the specification of eligibility criteria, the creation of hospital discharge guidelines and so on, have done little more than persuade many people that the problems of service fracture are so deep that nothing short of more wholesale reorganisation offers any prospect of remedy. However, one of the more hopeful aspects of the last generation of experimentation has been the experience of joint commissioning now incorporated into primary care. In the words of the White Paper,[16] the intention is to

> *better integrate primary and community health services and work more closely with social services on both planning and delivery. Services such as child health or rehabilitation where responsibilities have been split within the health service and where liaison with Local Authorities is often poor, will particularly benefit.*

Whether the return to joint planning, welded together with reorganised primary care and the possibility of reorganised social services, will be enough to crack the problems once and for all is not yet clear. But the experience of joint commissioning is worth examining because it does offer practical ways forward for PCGs to create a more effective and more integrated approach to care delivery.

Joint commissioning

There is no universally agreed definition of joint commissioning and one of the first tasks that PCGs and their partners need to establish is an agreed working definition of what they are trying to achieve by working together to commission services. As experience develops, so the working definition will change but unless there is some shared view at the outset the probability of failure and frustration is high. There are various definitions, which some agencies have found helpful and which can provide a starting point for reaching a shared view.

Gostick[17] defined collaborative commissioning as:

the process by which strategy is translated into action. Collaborative commissioning is the process by which two or more agencies share responsibility for that process equally for their mutual benefit ... it is the overarching activity whereby jointly agreed objectives are translated into action on the basis of shared vision and values.

The Department of Health guidance on joint commissioning, *An Introduction to Joint Commissioning*,[18] defined joint commissioning as:

the process when two or more commissioning agencies act together to co-ordinate their commissioning, taking joint responsibility for translating strategy into action, in order to achieve better outcomes for users and carers.

and the practical guidance issued in 1995[19] noted that:

Joint commissioning should be seen as both a strategic activity for agencies to share and discuss their overall perspectives and strategies, and as a more detailed problem solving tool for tackling specific difficulties.

Challis and Pearson[20] in their guide to local joint commissioning adopted the following definition:

... joint commissioning is the process of commissioning help and support within a local area for older people and their carers. It is a process which should involve a range of agencies, including health and social services, and users and carers. It is a process which requires networking, local needs assessment, creative approaches to meeting those needs, and contracting and purchasing. The aim is to produce more effective, more sensitive, more efficient and better co-ordinated care for people who need help.

Which agencies and organisations are part of the joint commissioning process? The potential cast list is very long indeed. Put in the most general terms the obvious candidates, in addition to the PCG, are users and carers, social services and housing authorities. However, such generalities do not take account of the different professional and occupational groups within each of the agencies. Clearly some decisions have to be made as to who is going to be a core participant in the joint commissioning process and who is to play a part as events unfold. This is why having a clear view of what joint commissioning is about is so important – it should help to focus attention upon who are the key players.

Not only is it important to be clear about which agencies are to be involved, it is also important to be clear about the level of membership needed. It is probably worth stating the obvious that there is a world of difference between commissioning a small pilot project and commissioning a major locality-wide service intended to be part of mainstream provision.[21] It is not just that the resources needed will be different, but so too will be the kind of expertise required. It will be worth thinking about the commissioning structures required. A core team at a strategic level might have an overview of the whole commissioning process, but for particular schemes or services it will be necessary to have specialised teams linked to the core group. The core group may develop the framework, both structures and processes, to which the project teams work.

Joint commissioning can be thought of as having a number of steps (*see* Figure 10.1).The rest of this chapter concentrates on the first three steps. Step 4, contracting and purchasing, should already be familiar territory to many staff in practices that were fundholding and other parts of the health services responsible for buying services.

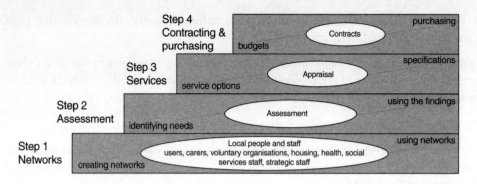

Figure 10.1:   Steps to joint commissioning.

Step 1: networks

The networking phase of joint commissioning has three stages: creating the network, which is where the basic work is done on deciding which agencies and individuals should be involved and in what capacity; networking itself, which is the process of people working together; and operating beyond the network, which entails spreading information into other relevant arenas and to agencies and individuals not actually part of the joint commissioning network.

The strategic/service level

CREATING THE NETWORK

At a strategic level the experience of pilot joint commissioning projects suggests that it is vital to get participants to own the work which is to be done. (The rest of this chapter draws heavily, but not exclusively, on the experience of joint commissioning projects established by the King's Fund; *see* Poxton.[21]) It will also be important that a clear steer is given to 'scheme' commissioning teams. In other words, it is as important with joint commissioning as with any other piece of complicated project work that the members of the network understand and are committed to the process and are clear about the outcomes they wish to see coming from the work. Experience also suggests that the involvement of user and carer organisations at this stage is vital so that plans can be rooted in experience and can be seen to be so rooted. A comment from a member of a local joint commissioning group underlines the importance of this:

> *in the beginning it was difficult to set up as no one really had any concrete idea of what joint commissioning meant. We also hadn't ever had contact with users and carers as such. Now listening to users' and carers' viewpoints and knowing how to do it has become part of the norm and so nothing is done without including them – so user and carer strategy is part of the services from square one.*

The commissioning team or group that 'represents' the wider network does need leadership, and that requires careful thought. This key role is not one that should pass by default to a particular individual. It will be better if the role is taken by someone who is particularly committed to success, has time to give to the tasks, and is not seen as completely aligned and committed to one agency above all others. It cannot be stressed enough that this kind of work requires time, so it is particularly important that time is not wasted through inefficiencies. The administration of the network needs to be worked out so that meetings are arranged properly, minutes are kept, action points progressed and so on. In other words, the network needs to be properly serviced.

NETWORKING

In working together at a strategic level, do keep in contact with projects at local level to keep up to date with the project progress; do not overburden local steering groups and networks with other agendas or initiatives decided on at strategic level, without first discussing it with the local networks and getting their agreement; do explain to local networks your role and purpose in attending any meetings and what information or lessons you are taking away with you; do not assume local members understand your role in your organisation and the implications of your presence at meetings.

USING THE NETWORK

Beyond the joint commissioning network itself do take lessons learned about joint commissioning to other groups / networks / meetings and do not compartmentalise joint commissioning experiences. It is very easy for joint commissioning groups to become insular as they develop knowledge and expertise. To overcome this, thought must be given to the ways in which staff and others are kept aware of developments. There are a variety of ways which might be useful – presentations, newsletters, open meetings, standing items on meeting agendas, etc. – and which should reduce the risk of duplication of effort and mistrust, and help to develop consensus.

The scheme/project level

CREATING THE NETWORK

People involved in joint commissioning at a strategic level are likely to understand that working productively across organisational boundaries is time-consuming, but at the more local levels and particularly with colleagues from some independent organisations or user and carer representatives it may not be self-evident. Two quotations from the Wiltshire pilot schemes make this plain:

> *In the beginning I was asked just to attend a couple of meetings to improve and develop respite care in the town, and now its been going for a year and a half and we have steering group meetings every month which last for about 2 hours, plus other things going on in between.* (Carer from one of the project sites)

And:

> *the users network ... chose to give considerable support to the King's Fund Project because it was suggested that this was the pattern of commissioning to come. We have found it very time-intensive.* (Convenor of the Wiltshire Users Network)

So, in identifying people to become part of a commissioning team it is important to make clear, as far as possible, what the time commitment is likely to be. It is also important to get clear the arrangements for expenses for involvement, to provide people with a proper briefing and to involve them in all aspects of the process of joint commissioning so that there is no suspicion that agencies or individuals are being marginalised or excluded from the 'real' meetings.

NETWORKING

Working together across professional and organisational boundaries provides fertile ground for misunderstanding as much as it provides an environment for sharing and exchanging knowledge and expertise. It is important that, as far as possible, professional labels and language do not inhibit free expression. Until trust has grown it will be necessary to be extra sensitive to the possibility that 'lay' members and others may feel at a disadvantage. Time must be allowed for clarifications and explanations of 'expert' knowledge or language. Efforts must be made to create opportunities, and to take advantage of opportunities, for people to contribute their personal expertise. However, it is also important that members do not lapse into the anecdotal and allow their personal experiences to override everything else. Persistence may be required to get points across. It is also very important of course that individual confidentiality is respected when particular examples are being used to illustrate or underline a point. None of this is easy as the following quotation recognises:

> *The wider remit a steering group has and the more professionals it embodies, the harder it is for a carer to feel at ease and willing to participate freely. Our steering group is very much one of local partnership and all members contribute freely and all decisions are made jointly.* (Representative of Carers Network)

It may be possible to organise the work of the team in such a way as to achieve some early successes. The effect of success on everyone is really quite dramatic. Not only is the success a worthy achievement in its own right, but it also provides individuals and agencies with a ready-made response to 'outsiders' who may be inclined to be sceptical or dismissive of the work being done and the time being taken to achieve it. This phenomenon has been noted frequently in pilot schemes and is typified by the response of a member of a users network:

> *I attended my first meeting with the King's Fund Project members with trepidation. I wasn't an older patient of the practice but an older member of the users network – a stranger. I need not have worried; I was made welcome, allowed to settle in and have been hooked ever since. An initiative being planned for improved care for older people by the health services and the social service working closely together at a local level, seemed great – and to me, dare I say, unusual! Everyone was enthusiastic, imaginative and willing to bounce ideas back and forth, and we all hope that some of that will come to fruition sooner rather than later; finances permitting of course – as usual. As all the ideas have stemmed from problems practice patients have discovered I'm sure they will be delighted to know what is afoot to help them keep going and able to stay at home as most older people want so much to do ... but it all takes time. Already it seems that the original acorn is growing and if it should flourish I hope that closer co-operation and joint commissioning between social services and health at local level will really take off in Wiltshire. It has been a real eye-opener for me to discover what can happen.*

However, equally important is not to use joint commissioning groups merely as a way of endorsing plans which have already been decided upon, or for 'rubber stamping'.

USING THE NETWORK

The value in spreading the experience of joint commissioning beyond the immediate network can be very great. For example, one of the members of a local steering group was also a co-ordinator of a transport scheme and was able to widen the remit of the scheme to meet some of the needs identified as part of the joint commissioning process.

Step 2: needs assessment for joint commissioning

The second step in joint commissioning is needs assessment, about which a great deal has been written.[22–24] The focus here, however, is on the special features of needs assessment when working with other agencies. It is probably worth saying that different agencies have approached needs assessment in different ways, so although there are a lot of data around, it is often not possible to use these data in a consistent and systematic fashion.

For example, in the social policy literature, need is closely connected to issues of equity and social justice and much attention is given to disentangling 'wants' from 'needs'. Doyal and Gough[25] propose the idea that need is no more than a preference shared by many people:

> *...social needs are demands which have been defined by society as sufficiently important to qualify for social recognition as goods or services which should be met by government intervention.*

The concept of health needs is particularly difficult to pin down because it is now generally agreed that health and social care overlap and that the boundaries are becoming even more blurred as more emphasis is placed on user and carer definitions and as the relationship between medical and social conditions comes to be better understood. Given that the notion of 'health' is now contested, it is hardly surprising that the character of health need is also somewhat fuzzy and becoming fuzzier.

However, practical joint commissioners do have to find ways towards working definitions of need which allow for services and schemes to be put in place. In general we can summarise the dominant perspectives as being of two main kinds:

- Person-based approaches by individuals, their carers or professionals, where the unit is an individual (case or care plans), a locality (GP practice or social service area), a population (national or regional), an age group (for example, people aged 75 and above), a medical or social condition (for example, people with dementia), an ethnic group (for example, Afro-Caribbean elders) or other group (for example, older women living alone).
- Service-based approaches, usually by professionals and service planners, where the unit is a service (for example, continuing care beds or home care or hip replacements) in a locality, a region or nationally. Services are usually classified according to the principal agency responsible for their delivery – health, social, financial, accommodation.

Whatever the level at which the assessment is being carried out and whatever the kind of need being examined, the basic materials for the assessment are likely to be similar. Demographic data will almost always be very important, of course, and so too will population estimates. Also important will be what might broadly be called prevalence data. The third major set of materials likely to be used are activity data, again defined broadly, which include the volume of service available, its origin and the intensity of use that is made of it.

Setting up a model for local needs assessment

The level at which the joint commissioners are working is obviously important when deciding what kind and how extensive the assessment should be. However, whatever the level there are some general principles that apply. It is, for example, sensible to collect together and make use of any available documents and information – population details, local services and provisions. In doing so it will probably be beneficial to carry out extensive user and carer consultations at the earliest stage and to cast the net wide to capture information from different sources. Although, in the interests of economy, it is also important to be clear about how you will use the information you collect.

Equally, it makes good sense to consider using methods that have been tried and tested elsewhere in similar exercises or projects.[24] The team may wish to consider what expert help may be needed and may decide to commission an external agency to carry out the assessment exercise rather than attempt to do it in-house.

Doing the local needs assessment

In conducting the needs assessment, the usual 'good housekeeping' rules for analysis apply. The people carrying out the assessment should be experienced; the methods to be used and the questions to be asked should be tested before the main study/analysis begins; enough time should be allowed for a rigorous analysis to be carried out; and, of course, individual and organisational confidentiality should be respected. It is also worth noting that a needs analysis should not raise unrealistic expectations in the respondents about what the exercise can achieve.

One example of needs research in a local joint commissioning project[26] took the form of a 'mapping and gapping' exercise to see if there was discrepancy between the respite provision and local needs. External researchers were commissioned to undertake the exercise. The areas identified to investigate were :

- to review current information held on the elderly population in the area
- to review current arrangements for involving users and carers in planning of local services
- to identify gaps in the services provision and assess whether needs were being met.

The method used was in-depth interviews with users, carers and providers, using a specifically designed questionnaire. The findings were the need for a sitting service, emergency respite and more flexible respite care.

Using the findings of the local needs assessment

Doing needs assessment is not an end in itself, it is there as a guide to planning and commissioning. Consequently it is important to circulate the findings of the exercise and feed the results back to the network members. It is also important to remember that the results do not always speak clearly for themselves, there will almost certainly be a need for interpretation.

Step 3: service design and specification

Step 3 is about designing schemes and services, designs based on needs assessment and the work of the network. Design alone is not sufficient to ensure that a service can be commissioned, the feasibility of the design and other options should be considered. Feasibility may be to do with practical, technical, financial and strategic feasibility.

Translating the findings into service possibilities

The experience of joint commissioning pilots has shown that the translation of needs analysis into practical service possibilities requires considerable creativity and ingenuity. If the assessment has focused on patient characteristics rather than on eligibility criteria for existing provision, the task is harder still but potentially one which allows greater scope for unfamiliar responses to what may be very familiar medical or social conditions. Given the brainstorming nature of this phase it may be worth considering setting up a small group to work on turning needs assessment into service possibilities that can be discussed with the network. It may also be useful to discuss the findings and the service/ scheme possibilities with provider units which may already have carried out some design work of their own or have experience of 'new' responses in other places. Discussing ideas with potential providers may also alert them to the need to gear up to make a response to some unmet need – a case of design discussions merging into implementation strategies.

Feasibility

The details of assessing the feasibility of particular scheme or service designs will, of course, depend on the particular features of the particular design. Perhaps it is necessary to say here that it may be that no new service is required but rather greater flexibility in the existing provision or simply more of the same. It is worth considering whether changes in existing services, e.g. more flexible or different hours, change in access or eligibility criteria, etc., can satisfy service shortfalls.

A very basic feasibility checklist would include such issues as the coverage and scope (numbers and geographical area) to be covered by the new service, that is:

- Is it to be intensive or extensive?
- What staff and skills would be required?
- How would patients/users access the scheme or service?
- What is the cost likely to be?
- Where might the funds come from?
- Which budgets?
- Is there 'private' demand for this service?
- Are there providers out there who are likely to be able to deliver the scheme or service?
- Is the design consistent with local and strategic priorities and plans?
- Is a development worker/project manager needed?

The checklist is a long one but one which will be familiar to many health and social care professionals. The feasibility work is probably best carried out by someone other than the joint commissioning team. If the project is a substantial one it may be worth considering whether outside help should be employed to undertake specified parts of the feasibility study.

It is important to keep the local network and users and carers informed at the planning and development phases to ensure that the proposal does not get too far away from the original objectives/identified needs. It is also important to be realistic about timescales so as not to undermine the confidence of the team and other members of the network. A pilot scheme to test feasibility can be very useful, not least because it does make clear that something is happening as a result of all the discussion and the research.

Specification

The service specification is at the heart of the joint commissioning process. It represents the culmination of design and feasibility and it also incorporates the best understanding of acceptable levels of quality and systems for monitoring its maintenance. The details will be scheme-specific, but once again there is now a substantial body of knowledge about how to write service specifications which can be drawn on from within the agencies.

Conclusion

PCGs have a crucial role in the realisation of the Government's plans for the NHS. A new ingredient of those plans is the emphasis on public health. The connection between health status and social condition is to be found on virtually every page of the Green Paper *Our Healthier Nation*.[27] It is precisely the kind of analysis which chimes with the ideas which have underpinned joint commissioning. As Christine Hancock, the General Secretary of the Royal College of Nursing commented, it is:

> *...an enormous opportunity to improve public health ... could bring an end to barriers between community, social, and hospital services.*

To help with the development of these important alliances, local authorities will be included in the duty of partnership to be placed on NHS bodies. It is regarded as vital that both health and local authorities take responsibility for their part in Health Improvement Programmes. Maybe the age of collaborative working is about to dawn, and maybe joint commissioning will be part of what makes it a reality at last.

References

1   Health Committee of the House of Commons (1993) *Report of the Health Committee of the House of Commons, 1992–93*. HMSO, London.

2   Clinical Standards Advisory Group (1998) *Community Health Care for Elderly People*. Stationery Office, London.

3   Huntingdon J (1981) *Social Work and General Medical Practice: collaboration or conflict?* Allen and Unwin, London.

4   Dongray M (1958) Social work in general practice. *BMJ*. **Nov 5**: 1220–3.

5   Goldberg EM, Neill J (1972) *Social Work in General Practice*. Allen and Unwin, London.

6   Marshall M, Hargreaves M (1979) So you want to try GP attachment? *Social Work Today*. **10**(42): 25–6.

7   Beales JG (1978) *Sick Health Centres and How To Make Them Better*. Pitman Medical, London.

8   Booth T (1981) Collaboration between the health and social services. *Policy and Politics*. **9**(1,2).

9   Glennerster H, Korman N, Marslen-Wilson F (1983) *Planning for Priority Groups*. Martin Robertson, London.

10   Wistow G, Fuller S (1983) *Joint Planning in Perspective: the NAHA Survey of Collaboration 1976–1982*. National Association of Health Authorities, Birmingham.

11   Challis L *et al.* (1987) *Joint Approaches to Social Policy*. Cambridge University Press, Cambridge.

12   Green DG (1986) Joint finance: an analysis of the reasons for its limited success. *Policy and Politics*, **14**(2): 209–20.

13   Nocon A (1990) Making a reality of joint planning. *Local Government Studies*. **16**: 55–67.

14   Audit Commission (1986) *Making a Reality of Community Care*. HMSO, London.

15   Griffiths Report (1988) HMSO, London.

16   Secretary of State for Health (1997) *The New NHS: modern, dependable*. The Stationery Office, London.

17   Gostick C (1993) *Collaborative Commissioning: issues and objectives*. North West Thames RHA.

18   Department of Health (1995) *An Introduction to Joint Commissioning*. Department of Health, London.

19   Department of Health (1995) *Practical Guide on Joint Commissioning for Project Leaders*. Department of Health, London.

20   Challis L, Pearson J (1996) *Getting in Step: a guide to practice based joint commissioning*. King's Fund and University of Bath.

21   Poxton R (1996) *Joint Approaches to a Better Old Age*. King's Fund, London.

22   Frankel S (1991) Health needs, healthcare requirements and the myth of infinite demand. *Lancet*. **337**.

23   Bradshaw J (1972) The social concept of need. *New Society*. **30 March**: 640–4.

24   Wilkin D, Hallam L, Doggett A-M (1992) *Measures of Need and Outcome for Primary Health Care*. Oxford University Press, Oxford.

25   Doyal L, Gough I (1984) A theory of human needs. *Critical Social Policy* **10**(4,1): 6–33.

26   Jelbert and Mitchell (1994).

27   Department of Health (1998) *Our Healthier Nation*. The Stationery Office, London.

Further reading

Audit Commission (1997) *The Coming of Age*. Audit Commission, London.

Challis L, Pearson J (1996) *Towards An Analysis of the Health and Social Care Needs of Older Londoners*. King's Fund and Oxford Brookes University.

Clayton S (1983) Social need revisited. *Journal of Social Policy*. **12**: 215–34.

Hawtin M, Hughes G, Percy-Smith J (1994) *Community Profiling: auditing social needs*. Open University Press, Buckingham.

House of Commons Health Committee (1993) *Sixth Report. Community Care: the way forward*, vol 1. HMSO, London.

Knapp M, Wistow G (1992) *Joint Commissioning for Community Care*. Conference Proceedings.

Knapp M, Wistow G (1993) Joint commissioning in community care. In: Department of Health, *Joint Commissioning: a slice through time*. DoH, London.

Pratt J (1995) *Practitioners and Practices: a conflict of values?* Radcliffe Medical Press, Oxford.

Raton L, Rose A, Smith CR (1974) Social workers and GPs. *Social Work Today*. **5**(16): 497–500.

Sheppard M (1992) Contact and collaboration with general practitioners: a comparison of social workers and community psychiatric nurses. *British Journal of Social Work*. **22**: 419–36.

Sidell M (1995) *Health in Old Age: myth, mystery and management*. Rethinking Ageing series. Open University Press, Buckingham.

CHAPTER ELEVEN

Public involvement

David Rowson

Tell me and I will forget
Show me and I will remember
Involve me and then I will care
(Old Chinese saying)

Increased participation by the public in decisions about local health services, and by individuals in their own care, has been a significant feature in the NHS over the past few years. It is possible to identify three levels of involvement[1]:

- **Accountability – public as citizens.** The NHS as a public service should be accountable. Accountability involves two processes: requiring those responsible for public services to give account of their actions and decisions; and establishing mechanisms through which they can be held to account for these actions. The process of giving account can be of value in its own right as a means of increasing dialogue between public officials and the public.
- **Organisational learning – public as service users (current, future or potential).** Feedback from users is an effective tool for monitoring service quality and standards and identifying improvements. This information provides commissioning intelligence. The public may also be involved in identifying need and in highlighting areas of current unmet need.
- **Individual empowerment.** Here the focus is on greater involvement of individuals in their own health and their own care and treatment.

The New NHS: modern, dependable[2] continues this process, asserting that greater public involvement in the NHS will rebuild confidence in the health service. Specific requirements have been set for primary care groups (PCGs) and public involvement will be one of their key areas for development.

An emerging force

Public involvement has been one element in the trend to increase the power of the consumer, relative to that of the producer or service provider, right across the public sector. Although there have been formal policy initiatives within the NHS, much of the development has been a result of bottom-up action by managers, clinicians and others within the health service.

Many within the NHS responded positively to shortcomings and limitations of existing methods for obtaining the views of local people. In many cases these were limited to ad hoc formal consultation and the 'public' restricted to the local community health council (CHC) as the statutory representative of user views in the NHS. Public meetings, often one-off, certainly unrepresentative of local people, and almost always on difficult and contentious issues such as closures of hospitals, were held only when necessary.

Many within the NHS were keen to move away from what was an adversarial relationship with the public and explore ways of entering into an ongoing dialogue with local people. Such a dialogue would give local decisions some legitimacy and, in seeking to explain and involve people in discussions about changes to services, help the management of change by giving local people more confidence in the reasons for change.

The pressure from the public themselves for more say has also contributed. Public involvement initiatives have indicated that the public want a say in decisions about their local services alongside professionals within the NHS, although they do accept that the final responsibility for decisions rests with the appropriate body.[3]

The public also acknowledge the resource limitations of the NHS. One of the conclusions of a National Consumer Council survey[4] was that the public are very aware of the need to balance the expectations they may have with the resources available.

Key legislative and policy initiatives have been:

- *Local Voices.*[5] Health authorities as purchasers of healthcare should take into account the views of local people in making decisions about what to purchase. Taking account of local people's views is a key function of health authorities. *Local Voices* states:

    ...their decisions (health authorities), should reflect, so far as practical, what people want, their preferences, concerns and values. Being responsive to local views will enhance the credibility of health authorities but, more importantly, is likely to result in services which are better suited to local needs and therefore more appropriate. There may of course be occasions when local views have to be over-ridden (e.g. on the weight of epidemiological, resource or other considerations) and in such circumstances, it is important that health authorities explain the reason for their decision.

- Patient's Charter (1992). The rights of individuals and the standards that could be expected when using the NHS set out. The emphasis is on the setting of targets and open reporting of performance against those standards. This process would enable the public to make comparisons of hospital performance on aspects such as waiting lists, and to make choices about where to have their treatment.

- Freephone health information service. The aim of the health information service is to provide information to the public, as a means of enabling them to become more active in relation to issues concerning their own healthcare and treatment and in matters relating to the development of healthcare policies and services.[6]
- Patient Partnership Strategy, which has four overall aims:
  - At the level of individual patient care, to promote user involvement in their own care, as active partners with professionals and to enable patients to become informed about their treatment and care and to make informed decisions and choices about it if they wish.
  - At the level of overall service development, to contribute to the quality of health services by making them more responsive to the needs and preferences of users, and to ensure that users have the knowledge, skills and support to enable them to influence NHS service policy and planning.

A programme of action was set out for taking the strategy forward at the national and local levels of the NHS.[7]

The New NHS: modern, dependable

The White Paper seeks the continued development of public involvement as a means of rebuilding confidence in the NHS:

> *The Government expects Health Authorities to play a strong role in communicating with local people and ensuring public involvement in decision making about the local health service ... the maxim is simple, the NHS as a public service for local communities, should be both responsive and accountable.*

The White Paper includes specific proposals for public involvement, including the first national survey of patient and user experience of the NHS, involvement of local communities in the development of Health Improvement Programmes (HImPs) and taking account of patient experiences in the new national framework for performance.[2]

The primary care group response

HSG 98/139 sets out the following requirements of PCGs:

- plans should be developed for the early, systematic and continuous involvement of users and the public
- PCGs should be able to demonstrate how in carrying out their role they have involved users and the public

- PCGs should provide feedback to users and the public on the outcome of their involvement.

All PCG boards will include a lay person to ensure they are more representative of the local community they serve.[8]

Rather than proscribe a single method of taking forward public involvement, what is suggested below is a framework within which the PCG can formulate its approach. In developing the framework there are two overriding considerations:

- the need to achieve organisational commitment
- the need to ensure the organisation has the capacity.

Organisational commitment

The successful development of public involvement will of course depend on the PCG's commitment. The requirement to open up to the public is challenging. It challenges management and clinician hegemony and involves subjecting ideas and proposals to scrutiny that some professionals within the NHS will find uncomfortable.

Top-down imposition through requirements set by national guidance are all very well but can lead to a minimalist 'box-ticking' approach to public involvement. What is more important to its success is that the organisation has the will to do it and sees it as a key part of its activities. Public involvement should become part of the fabric of the PCG – it should be part of the way you do things.

A board member should take responsibility for the development of public involvement within the PCG and have the lead for overseeing its development. It should also be part of the Chief Executive's core responsibilities and written into their job description and any individual objectives set as part of the performance review targets. The board member responsible should adopt the role of 'agent provocateur', identifying opportunities for public involvement and challenging others to build it into projects such as service reviews. This lead role will also entail keeping up-to-date with developments in public involvement and acting as a point of contact for local groups.

The PCG should include a reference to public involvement in any mission or purpose statement it produces. Not only is organisational commitment to doing the work essential, but also a commitment to use the findings. This does not mean that decisions will be changed simply on the basis of what the public have said, but there needs to be commitment to taking these views into account alongside those of other stakeholders.

Organisational capacity

Public involvement will require a substantial investment of resources – time, people and money. The range of public involvement techniques will mean that that the PCG is likely to require additional support from external sources. Links should be established with the health authority lead (all are likely to have a lead for patient partnership initiatives). Local trusts are also likely to have lead staff for patient partnership initiatives and may have carried out initiatives that have drawn on patient experiences. Clinical audit departments may, for example, have some expertise in methods for surveying patients. There may also be potential partnerships with local authorities who have interests in developing initiatives to promote local dialogue, particularly methods to identify needs in local communities.

Working with other PCGs on particular initiatives may also be appropriate. For example, the service provided by a particular trust may be subject to public involvement. The findings from this work will benefit patients of other PCGs, so it seems appropriate to carry out such work in partnership.

Finally, it is inevitable that much public involvement work will require specialist input. PCGs will need to purchase such support from research organisations and independent researchers, many of whom have specialist knowledge of the public sector. Local universities will also be keen to work jointly on initiatives and provide expertise on research initiatives. It may also be possible to 'piggy-back' on the work of others, for example voluntary groups or self-help groups who may have undertaken initiatives or collected evidence of patient experiences. The CHC, the statutory representative of users in the NHS, may have task groups monitoring particular services and have special rights to enter hospitals for the purpose of keeping a check on standards of care.

A policy for involvement

The commitment to public involvement should be stated in a policy adopted by the PCG. The policy should cover:

- statement of commitment
- broad definition of 'the public'
- why users are being involved
- how users will be involved
- principles which should govern user involvement, e.g. equal opportunities, feedback on decisions etc.[9]

Who are 'the public'?

So far 'the public' has been used as though PCGs are serving an homogeneous group. In reality there are many different publics and arrangements for public involvement should acknowledge this. Examples include:

- **Community Health Councils** are the statutory representatives of consumers within the NHS. CHCs have specific rights to be consulted about changes to local services. They also carry out a monitoring of local services and have rights to enter hospitals to check on standards of care. CHCs may have working groups focusing on specific services.

- **Voluntary organisations.** In any area there will be a plethora of user groups, self-help groups and other forms of voluntary organisations representing the interests of service users or people affected by a particular condition or illness, representing carers or particular sections of the local community. Voluntary organisations provide a captive audience for dialogue and an effective means of obtaining the views of particular groups of people.
- **Service users** can be divided into past, present and future/potential users.
- **Local opinion formers.** These include local politicians (councillors and MPs), editors of local newspapers, other members of the local media, community representatives (e.g. religious leaders).
- **Different local populations** can be distinguished by age, sex, socio-economic or ethnic background, geographical location, etc. The target 'public' will depend on the issue under scrutiny.

The essentials of the framework

In developing the framework it is essential that the PCG has an agreed understanding of what it means by public involvement. In practice, public involvement has become the collective term for a range of initiatives.

Sherry Arnstein developed the *Ladder of Participation* as a guide for clarifying different levels of participation (*see* Figure 11.1).[10] The ladder highlights that as one moves up to the top three rungs power begins to shift from professionals and organisations to people. However, even at the lower levels, such as informing, people are beginning to have the opportunity to take some control.

The ladder is a useful tool for helping PCGs to develop their approach to public involvement. PCGs should use a spectrum of activities, employing specific methods appropriate

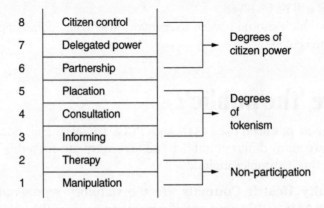

Figure 11.1:   The ladder of participation.

to the issue being discussed. At some point the provision of information will be the appropriate mechanism, at others consultation. The range of mechanisms needed by the PCG should cover the following:

- Listening – ensure arrangements are in place to enable the voice of local people to be heard.
- Informing – provide sufficient easily understood information to support a local, informed debate.
- Discussing – ensure there is an opportunity to discuss proposals, and that decisions ultimately take account of local views.
- Reporting – ensure decisions are reported back, including feedback and responses from public involvement initiatives.
- Ongoing dialogue – public involvement should be part of an ongoing dialogue with local people not a one-off exercise which runs the risk of being regarded as a PR stunt.

The commissioning cycle

The importance of an ongoing dialogue with the public has been emphasised. The commissioning cycle (*see* Figure 11.2) presents opportunities for public involvement.

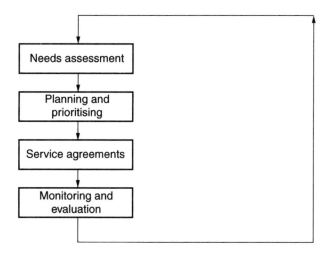

Figure 11.2:   The commissioning cycle.

Needs assessment

Involving people in needs assessment can help to identify gaps in service and unmet needs. For example, dialogue with particular ethnic community groups may provide reasons why a particular sector of the community makes less use of a service. Involving people at this stage in the commissioning process could help to ensure services are more appropriate to the needs of local communities. Services which more appropriately meet the needs of users may lead to better take-up.

Planning and priority setting

At this point in the commissioning process involving people is more complex and one of the most contentious aspects of involvement is that different people will obviously place different values on services or treatments. The priority given to one service over another will be influenced by whether there has been direct experience and knowledge of a particular service and the values intrinsic to an individual.

The pressure on NHS resources and the need to set priorities – or more precisely the need to declare some services low priority (IVF for example) – has led to the development of techniques which allow exploration of issues in more depth. Public involvement work has increasingly focused on the values and criteria used by health authorities for determining which services should be low priority. Cambridge and Huntingdon Health Authority, for example, used a citizen jury process to discuss the setting of values and criteria to be used for deciding whether a procedure or treatment should be classified as low priority. City and Hackney Health Authority asked local residents to rank services to determine high and low priority care and treatments.

One point of public involvement initiatives such as this is to bring into the open priority setting; some health authorities have set up priority forums and public views are sought as part of this.

Service plans

Local people should have the opportunity to discuss and comment on draft plans. At this stage the public involvement process will focus on the provision of information and is likely to involve public meetings. Consideration should also be given to the style of any documentation published. A commitment to involve and inform local people will not be met by the production of inaccessible documents. For example, you will need to consider the level of detail. Service plans will often have to meet the needs of a variety of audiences, but the language and level of detail necessary for those within the NHS will often be inappropriate for the public. Consideration should be given to publishing summary versions and perhaps working with the local media on feature articles. Feedback can be encouraged by including a questionnaire in the service plan document or by inviting responses from readers of the feature article.

Consideration will also need to be given to printing the documents in different languages to meet the needs of communities for whom English is a second language.

Service agreements and specifications

Public involvement at this point in the commissioning cycle should focus on the development of service standards. The views of users could be useful for:

- identifying key aspects of services for which standards should be set
- suggesting quality improvements in services.

Monitoring and evaluation of services

Opportunities for public involvement at this point are focused on feedback on the public's experiences of services. Opportunities should be established for users to feedback complaints and suggestions on service improvements.

Health outcomes

Following a particular course of treatment or procedures, the views of users can be obtained to assess the practical impact of treatments or services on their lifestyle (for example, when were they able to return to work?).

The agenda may appear overwhelming but PCGs can build their public involvement activities on to existing activities.

Public meetings

PCGs are required to hold their board meetings in public. Regular board meetings provide an opportunity for informing the public and reporting on decisions. The Board should consider inviting representatives from interest groups to make presentations on specific issues. Board meetings could perhaps focus on particular service issues from time to time or be turned into open forums to allow interested people to put views forward.

Even if public meetings are poorly attended there is likely to be interest from the media so there are opportunities to convey messages through them. The Board should consider issues of accessibility to their public meetings and consider holding the meetings in different geographical locations and at different times.

Complaints systems

All GP practices are required to have a complaints process in place. Complaints can provide an indication of a service shortfall or failing. Access to trust complaints can be used positively for developing quality and challenging service providers to make improvements.

Freephone health information service

All health authorities are required to secure the provision of a freephone health information service. Most health information services (HIS) will provide regular reports on enquiries by type of question and geographical location. Information such as this could be made available to PCGs to help identify issues of concern in local areas. The HIS can also provide a useful point for distribution of information about the PCG and the decisions it makes.

Local media

It will be essential for PCGs to develop a communications strategy, a key element of which will be relationships with the local media. The media provide a channel of communication to a relatively large audience. The media are always keen to cover local health stories so a steady stream of press releases will be an effective means of informing local people.

Publicity and information

The PCG should ensure that information about its work is available to local people. The need to ensure information is accessible both in format and content is essential, including meeting the needs of those whose first language is not English. PCGs may wish to consider publishing their own community newsletter.

In addition to the media above, information could be made available through local authority newsletters and voluntary organisation newsletters. In producing information, opportunities for feedback should be given to recipients.

Tools and techniques

The following list is not exhaustive but represents a sample of the more common techniques in use within the NHS. There are many different tools and techniques and many of those below can be adapted to fit local circumstances.

Health panels

Health panels are mainly used to inform planning and prioritising decisions requiring a wider population view. Typically panels are made up of between eight and ten people and are a representative sample (age, sex, location, race, etc.) of the area they are drawn from. Panels meet for a number of sessions to discuss set topics and give their views.

Box 11.1:   Somerset health panels

These were set up as part of a consultation programme, the long-term aims of which were '...to build a consensus on the values to be used to guide health resource allocation'.

Eight panels were set up across an area of Somerset, with 12 members on each panel. Panels meet three times per year and all panels discuss the same issues. Topics discussed have included:
- Should smokers be offered coronary artery bypass operations?
- Should people be able to choose treatment from another health authority if it is unavailable in Somerset?
- Should the health authority pay for intensive treatment for people with terminal cancer and less than six months to live?
- Should IVF be available on the NHS in Somerset?[11]

A variation on the above are postal panels. A larger representative sample of people (e.g. 500) may be sent questionnaires on particular issues. These panels can be useful for reaching those groups of people who may not attend a meeting or find it difficult to attend a session.

Box 11.2:   Bedfordshire local health comment groups

County-wide local health comment group of approximately 2000 people recruited to represent the demographic profile of the seven localities in the health authority. The group acts as a link between Bedfordshire and each of the localities to communicate information about health in the county and advises and comments on healthcare services.[12]

Rapid appraisal

Rapid appraisal is a technique used to provide qualitative information about needs and priorities for change, usually focused on a particular geographical area (e.g. areas that are relatively deprived). The process is carried out by a multidisciplinary team who have knowledge of a particular area. This team interviews key members of the community to

---

Box 11.3:   Lambeth, Southwark and Lewisham

Rapid appraisal used as part of a project to enhance the quality of out-of-hours provision in the district.[13]

---

gather views in a rapid but systematic way. The aims of rapid appraisal are to identify common priorities and needs, translate the findings into action and to build an ongoing relationship between service providers, purchasers and the community.[9]

Citizens' jury

A citizens' jury is an approach to public involvement developed in Germany and brought to this country by the Institute for Public Policy Research (IPPR).[14] The approach is particularly appropriate for involving the wider public in decision making, particularly over service priorities. The jury consists of 12 members of the public, who are paid to attend as a jury member for four days and then make a decision on a question. During the process, 'witnesses' are called to give evidence on specific subjects and are questioned by the jurors. Compared with other models of public involvement juries allow for more information to be provided and more deliberation and discussion.

Box 11.4:   IPPR pilot juries

The IPPR funded three pilot citizens' juries as part of a UK Pilot Project:

- Cambridge and Huntingdon HA: rationing (values and criteria underpinning decisions about low priorities and involvement of the public in rationing decisions)
- Kensington, Chelsea and Westminster with Riverside Mental Health Trust: two juries to consider how mental health services could be improved
- Walsall: improvements to palliative care services

Focus groups

Focus groups are in-depth discussion groups of between six and ten people which are focused around a specific set of issues or topics. The discussion is facilitated by an independent researcher and usually an observer, who will take notes of the discussions. Focus groups are useful for identifying a range of issues around a specific subject, participants prompting each other as the discussion develops. The ability of focus groups to identify a range of issues means that they may also be used as part of the process of designing a questionnaire/survey.

Box 11.5: Berkshire Health Authority

The health authority has used focus groups on a range of topics:

- What makes a good cancer service? Focus groups with past and present patients asked to identify the key elements of a good cancer service as part of local implementation of Calman–Hine[15]
- Sensitivity to a range of policy options: a series of representative focus groups were held across the health authority area to test reactions to different scenarios for allocating resources[16]
- Methods of communication: focus groups to identify preferred methods of communication to be used by the health authority. Attitudes to health authority literature were also tested[17]

Surveys and interviews

Interviews may be:

- *Structured*: questions are asked in a standardised form from a structured questionnaire
- *Semi-structured*: questions are open-ended but define the area to be explored.

Box 11.6: Public perception of cancer services and cancer care provided in Buckinghamshire

Aim of the survey was to identify the attitudes, beliefs and information needs of the Buckingham population regarding cancer, its treatment, screening and health promotion. Face-to-face interviews were held with 1000 people[18]

References

1 NHS Executive, Institute of Health Service Management and The NHS Confederation (1998) *In the Public Interest: developing a strategy for public participation in the NHS.* Department of Health, London.

2 Secretary of State for Health (1997) *The New NHS: modern, dependable.* Stationery Office, London.

3 Barker J (1995) *Local NHS Health Care Purchasing and Prioritising from the Perspective of Bromley Residents – a Qualitative Study.* Bromley Health.

4 National Consumer Council (1998) *Consumer Concerns 1998: a consumer view of health services.* National Consumer Council, London.

5   NHS Management Executive (1992) *Local Voices: the views of local people in purchasing for health.* NHSE, London.

6   NHS Executive (1995) *Provision of the National Freephone Health Information Service.* HSG(95)44. NHSE, London.

7   NHS Executive (1996) *Patient Partnership Strategy: building a collaborative strategy.* NHSE, London.

8   NHS Executive (1998) *Developing Primary Care Groups.* HSG(98)139. Department of Health, London.

9   Fleming B, Golding L (1997) *Briefing Papers: involving users,* vol 1. Soundings Research, Birmingham.

10 Arnstein S (1969) *A Ladder of Citizen Participation in the USA.* Originally published in the *Journal of the American Institute of Planners.* **July**: 216–25.

11 Richardson A (1996) *Illiciting Public Views in Somerset.* Somerset Health Authority.

12 Bedfordshire Health Authority (1994) *Local Health Comment Groups.* Bedfordshire HA.

13 Dale J, Shipman C, Lacock L, Davies M (1996) Creating a shared vision of out of hours care: using rapid appraisal methods to create an interagency, community orientated, approach to service development. *BMJ.* **312**.

14 Coote A, Lenaghan J (1997) *Citizens' Juries: theory into practice.* Institute for Public Policy Research, London.

15 Berkshire Health Authority (1996) *What Makes a Good Cancer Service?* Berkshire HA.

16 Berkshire Health Authority (1995) *Public Attitude Study: assessing public attitudes. Various Options.* Berkshire HA.

17 Berkshire Health Authority (1994) *Public Attitude Study: planned changes in health care provision and methods of communication.* Berkshire HA.

18 Social and Market Strategic Research Ltd (1997) *Public Perception of Cancer Services and Cancer Care Provided in Buckinghamshire and Other Health Issues.* Buckinghamshire Health Authority.

Further reading

Barker J, Bullen M, de Ville J (1997) *Reference Manual for Public Involvement.* Bromley Health, West Kent Health Authority and Lewisham, Southwark and Lambeth Health Authority.

Barnes M (1997) *The People's Health Service.* NHS Confederation, London.

College of Health (1994) *Consumer Audit Guidelines (a guide for health professionals on College of Health Consumer Audit methods).* College of Health, London.

Lewthwaite J, Haffenden S (1997) *Patients Influencing Purchasers.* NHS Confederation and Longterm Medical Conditions Alliance, London.

CHAPTER TWELVE

The contribution of nurses, commissioning and fundholding GPs

Lorna Hipkin, Michael Dixon and Peter Smith

PART 1

What community nurses have to offer primary care groups

Lorna Hipkin

The community nurse in the context of primary care group development

Community nurses are an integral part of primary care groups (PCGs). Alongside GP colleagues in the PCG, the White Paper *The New NHS: modern dependable*,[1] offers them '...the opportunity to deploy resources and savings to strengthen local services and ensure that patterns of care best reflect their patients' needs'.

This gives community nurses a legitimate role in local decision making and responsibility for ensuring that the functions of PCGs are delivered.[2] Nurses hold this responsibility at Board level, as advisors to the Board and as practitioners working within the PCG.

The PCG provides the opportunity to develop an organisation that can function with equal 'partners' and that can learn and develop through sharing skills, knowledge, networks and workloads. It should be able to develop the further skills and expertise required to achieve the objectives of the PCG through multidisciplinary skills audit and shared education programmes.[3]

The lack of 'shared objectives amongst the different professionals involved'[4] has been highlighted in many primary healthcare teams leading to a lack of co-ordinated care across a practice population. PCGs should be in a position to build on such findings and others. In doing so, they should be able to agree objectives that:

* assist in the determination of what needs to be done
* identify the skills and expertise required
* ensure effective communication systems
* determine ways of working.[5]

Community nurses have a role to play in designing and developing the PCG organisation just as they do in ensuring that its functions are fulfilled. Antrobus and Brown (1997)[6] proposed '...that unless nurses understand and engage in debate around the ... commissioning function in health care, nursing's capacity to influence the future development of patient services will be severely limited'.

PCGs give nurses that opportunity – influencing healthcare and influencing the structures that are responsible for deciding and determining that care. This requires a sound contribution from community nurses.

The community nurse contribution to PCGs

Local knowledge

Community nurses have tremendous local knowledge.[7] They are connected into formal and informal healthcare systems in a local area. As such, they are able to assess change in delivery of service or care and its impact on patients. They are sensitive to changes within the community and have access to the views of the community, including individual or client group expectations, experiences and perceptions.

They tend to have credibility in local communities and may be seen as more approachable than medical colleagues. They may also develop strong links with women in communities who undertake key roles, such as carers[8] or informal opinion leaders.

Such local knowledge adds to that of other colleagues and other sources. This knowledge is important in:

* providing rapid enviromental feedback regarding possible or actual change affecting the population that may require the PCG to adapt its commissioning strategy or ways of working
* considering how services are functioning

- assessing whether objectives are appropriate
- encouraging the public to become actively involved in healthcare commissioning.

Community nurses are in an ideal position to work closely with the public on self-care initiatives and in working to share knowledge, support and power, acting '...as facilitators who help people to take charge of their own health.'[9] Such a role is not confined to employed or 'attached' community nurses but will include community psychiatric nurses and specialist nurses.

Networks

Local knowledge is obtained through strong networks. Networks are established for patient benefit and are dynamic. They provide contacts with other parts of the healthcare system and other agencies. They also act as channels to assist in updating on professional and practice change and development.

Wider networks are established by specialist nurses, those working in areas such as diabetes, complex paediatric care, or with client groups such as the homeless or travellers.

Specialist nurse advice will have greater relevance across the wider population base of the PCG. Access to networks and specialist nurse input will:

- assist PCG development and learning
- allow access to a greater knowledge base, expertise and advice for patient benefit
- provide direct advice on issues such as infection control, immunisation, and specialist nursing care
- encourage liaison, support and training between specialist nurses and PCGs.

Needs assessment and profiles

Information is collected by community nurses for statistics, to assist planning and for the formation of local health profiles. Such information should assist PCGs as they put together local databases.

Health profiling is an approach that nurses have taken to assess local need. The approach is strongly advocated by many nurses and supported through professional education programmes.

Compiling profiles is a key means of increasing awareness of population needs, needs assessment and need for service change, and has helped to develop local alliances and priority setting within nursing workloads.[10]

There have been concerns about the validity of data and problems with verifying it because of limited access to GP and health authority data. Debates about measurement of needs have affected confidence in profiling as have difficulties in implementation of change.

Community nurses will bring to PCGs the skills that have been developed in profiling and epidemiological knowledge which will be invaluable as PCGs develop approaches to health needs assessment. With a wider base of multi-agency information the profiling approach should reach its next stage with findings being applied to change programmes to benefit the public's health.

Ways of working

Applying 'old' skills

Community nurses work at many levels with many agencies. The skills used to undertake their work include:[7]

- assessment
- evaluation
- problem solving
- decision making
- priority setting, within time, financial and staffing constraints
- networking
- clinical skills
- and many others.

Although this is obvious, it is important that the use of these skills is recognised and appreciated because, applied in a different setting, they will form the basis for sound commissioning.

Partnership and collaborative working with social services is a crucial part of the way nurses work in the community. Links with social services will be very important for PCGs. As nurses tend to have closer relationships with social services, they will be able to assist the PCG in working together across agency and geographical boundaries.

Acquiring new skills

Recent years have seen changes in the ways that community nurses work, with integration of nursing teams and self-management of teams. They appear to have created some positive results for nurses although further work is needed on evaluation.[11]

Some community nurses are thus used to significant changes in the way they work. Skills developed to adapt to these changes have included budgetary responsibility, facilitation of the team and negotiation. These new skills are highly relevant for the new healthcare agenda.

Teamworking is an integral part of the community nurse's role. The PCG is bigger than a team but collaborative working across the extended nursing team could reap very positive results for patients if expertise and skills are used as criteria for determining input. The size of PCGs should allow for robust planning and development of specialist expertise and an appropriate workforce to meet changing patient needs.

Clinical knowledge and professional practice

Community nurses' clinical knowledge continuously develops with changes in the complexity of patient care, healthcare settings and length of stay. Such knowledge is available to PCGs to form the basis of advice and to provide services commissioned from local primary healthcare teams.

Community nurses are required to update professional knowledge and practice as part of the renewal of registration. This focus on professional practice, supported by professional education programmes, increasingly emphasises reflective, evaluative and research-based practice, peer assessment and clinical audit. These professional activities plus the Code of Professional Conduct [12] provide the basis for a useful approach to clinical governance in PCGs.

Getting the best from the nursing contribution

Valuing the contribution

There has to be respect for and recognition of the value of the contribution. Nurses can undervalue their contribution, seeing commissioning as medically or managerially led and needing a different set of skills than their own.

Realising the potential and power

Nurses' views are not automatically sought and nurses can be reticent in offering them. Their contribution to fundholding was sporadic and unsystematic,[6] hence there is no ready model for PCGs to apply. Therefore an opportunity arises for nurses to recognise their potential and realise it through mutual support and encouragement from other professional colleagues, nurse leaders in PCGs and elsewhere, and educationalists.

Nurses have real power[13] in PCGs not gained through predetermined status but through their ability to influence, to network, to use and acquire skills and knowledge, and now through their legitimate involvement in determining change and use of resources through commissioning. This is a powerful position indeed.

Developing agreed new ways of working

Acknowledging that PCGs are not replica primary healthcare teams and building a different kind of organisation will be important in removing actual or perceived barriers to nurses' contribution.

Hierarchical relationships are inappropriate for PCGs, with their requirement for multidisciplinary and multi-agency assessment, planning and action. However, the dangers of nurses' input being ignored or excluded by their employers – the GPs – is a particular concern for practice nurses and needs to be resolved as part of the Board's role in establishing ways of working. The role played by community trusts will also be crucial in encouraging and assisting nurses' contribution and should be explicitly agreed with the health authority and PCG Board.

Summary

There is a substantial and significant role for community nurses in PCGs, whether at board level or advising the Board, their colleagues in primary healthcare teams or the board level nurse.

Their contribution to PCGs includes a wide range of skills which are applied to clinical care and ways of working, and will now be applied to commissioning.[7] Local knowledge, the process of gaining it and its application is a key contribution from nurses, alongside clinical practice, approaches to needs assessment, joint working and professional development.

References

1   Secretary of State for Health (1997) *The New NHS: modern, dependable.* Stationery Office, London.

2   NHS Executive (1998) *Developing Primary Care Groups.* HSC 1998/139. NHSE, London.

3   Wilson T, Butler F, Watson M (1998) *Defining the Education and Training Needs of Primary Care Groups.* Public Health Resource Unit, Oxford.

4   West M, Poulton BC (1997) A failure of function: teamwork in primary care. *Journal of Interprofessional Care.* **11**(2): 205–16.

5   Mullins L (1996) *Management and Organisational Behaviour.* Pitman Publishing, London.

6   Antrobus S, Brown S (1997) The impact of the commissioning agenda upon nursing practice – a proactive approach to influencing health policy. *Journal of Advanced Nursing.* **25**: 309–15.

7   Hipkins L (1998) *Nurses and Commissioning.* A study of skills that nurses bring to and that nurses need for commissioning. Anglia and Oxford Regional Office.

8   Webb C (1986) *Feminist Practice in Women's Health Care.* Wiley, Chichester.

9   Nakajima KW (1992) More than ever we need nurses. *World Health.* **Sept–Oct**: 3.

10 Billings JR, Cowley S (1995) Approaches to community needs assessment: a literature review. *Journal of Advanced Nursing.* **22**: 721–30.

11 Young L, Poulton B (1997) Integrated nursing teams can influence locality commissioning. *Primary Health Care.* **7**(10): 8–10.

12 Code of Professional Conduct for the Nurse, Midwife and Health Visitor. United Kingdom Central Council.

13 Johnson G, Scholes K (1993) *Exploring Corporate Strategy.* Prentice Hall, New York.

PART 2

Commissioning GPs and locality groups – what can they tell us about future primary care groups?

Michael Dixon

GP commissioners come to primary care groups (PCGs) with a strong message as well as practical expertise. Fundholders and total purchasing projects were able to innovate within the limits of what was then government policy. GP commissioners effectively demanded a complete 'rewrite'. They were responding to an overwhelming call from grass roots professionals and locality groups, which had reacted to a system that had excluded local professionals from any planning role. It was a system that had produced an NHS where inequality and unfairness were widespread and there were divisions between GPs and between them, other primary care professionals, health authorities and trusts. That GP commissioners were able to change the national agenda at all is perhaps an important lesson for primary care professionals involved in future PCGs. That is to say grass roots professionals should not underrate their expertise in formulating a workable system as well making it a success.

Commissioning GPs expressed their aims in *Restoring the Vision*,[1] a document that had been commissioned by the Government shortly before the White Paper was published. Their aims were:

> *To develop a comprehensive NHS that is fair to those who use it and those who work within it, efficient and effective in its use of resources; sensitive to the needs of individuals and communities; and openly accountable for its actions.*

It is no coincidence that this is the vision for PCGs outlined in the White Paper.[2] This emphasises the importance of health as something that goes on beyond the surgery walls and which must involve the whole community. The message is that you get the best out of people and the best deal for patients when they are co-operating rather than when they are in conflict and that you must have ground rules of fairness for both professionals and patients. Commissioning GPs may have provided the rhetoric – did their locality groups tell us anything useful about future PCGs?

Doctors working with doctors

Like future PCGs, locality commissioning groups covered specific geographical areas and included all doctors within a given locality. Those doubting whether GPs will be able to work together in future PCGs should take heart from 175 locality groups, which are detailed on the NHS Primary Care Group Alliance website.[3] Many started as disparate groups of GPs but found that a successful formula has been to develop an atmosphere of mutual respect and trust and a feeling of group ownership. An essential part of this has been inclusiveness – not isolating rebels but valuing them, understanding them and involving them, as the most avid dissenters often become the most active supporters in the end. The first job of any PCG will be to get the group dynamics right – textbooks[4] may help, but personal contact with experienced locality commissioners may be most useful.

Leadership

Locality commissioning groups did not evolve because 50 or 60 doctors thought spontaneously that they would be a good idea, but because a number of leaders arose all over the country to get the process on its feet. They have learnt to be 'gentle' leaders with a democratic mandate but no hierarchy, where inspiration, persuasion and creating unity of purpose was everything. Some of the locality commissioning group lead GPs have been employed part time by their health authorities and have learnt to merge their role as democratic leader with that of an accountable officer who has to deliver the goods. It is a balancing act that board members and leaders in PCGs will need to carry out wisely, especially when resources are scarce and unreasonable demands are being made both from the top and the bottom. In many groups, a GP lead has worked with a locality manager from the health authority as part of a 'matched pair'. These have created a strong manager/GP bond, which has tempered the centralist and hierarchical agenda of the manager, while providing the GP with a better idea of some of the complex accountability issues that health authorities have always faced and GPs have historically tried to avoid. In future PCGs it will be particularly important that the personalities of chief officer and PCG chair (which will in most cases be a GP) are matched in the sense of being compatible rather than the same. The ideal should be to formulate a relationship of respect, trust and hopefully liking but which allows a frisson of creative tension and open debate. If GP and manager provide too much of a united front then there is a danger that those around them will feel that they are being 'stitched up'.

Working with other professionals

Commissioning was started by GPs but both of the books by those involved in locality commissioning[4,5] emphasised both the desirability as well as the inevitability of involving other primary care professionals. Some locality groups started the ball rolling and are contactable on the NHS Alliance website.[3] In particular, some groups (e.g. Langbaurgh Coast Commissioning Group) have successfully included nurses and managers on their boards; some have included practice managers (e.g. Mid Devon Commissioning Group), while others (e.g. Small Heath Commissioning Group, Birmingham) have involved social services.

Involving the public

The key to success in PCGs will be proper public involvement. This is not only because they should be democratically involved in making local health decisions. It is also because the involvement of the public in rationing decisions will support the work of the health professionals, who may then feel less isolated. An unexpected development in locality commissioning has been the discovery that the public have an important potential role in providing services, as a successful locality initiative in promoting self-care can free up professional resources for those in greatest need. Some locality groups (e.g. Newcastle West Primary Care Group) have developed innovative ways of including the public, such as employing a community worker whose job is to find out what the public really think, want and need. Medics are traditionally shy of both patient views and the media but the experience of locality commissioners is that both can be very powerful allies in the commissioning process and contributors in the process of provision.

Involving health authorities

Locality commissioners were unlike fundholders in that if they had a poor relationship with the health authority then nothing happened. Locality commissioning groups therefore bring a lot of experience about how to work with health authorities simply because they were only able to achieve anything when they had gained their support. Some lead GPs in locality commissioning groups sat on subcommittees of health authorities (like future PCGs) and in some cases lead GPs became an intrinsic part of the health authority itself. Such arrangements allowed locality commissioning groups an extended role in planning for their localities while being collectively integrated at health authority level with other groups in very much the same way as PCGs will be. Access to public health at health authority level gave groups the necessary evidence, epidemiological data and assessment of needs, which they required to make locality health strategies. Some, though still in an advisory role, had considerable influence over health authority purchasing decisions and one or two were given indirect control over contracts by having their wishes included in the health authority purchasing intentions.[6] They found that if their relationship with their health authority was particularly good then it became less necessary to hold a budget in order to influence purchasing decisions – indeed unnecessary if health authorities were able to considerably sharpen up their purchasing efficiency. This did not, of course, exclude the desirability of holding budgets (upheld in *Restoring the Vision*[1]) for virement purposes where a group was successful in managing demand in particular areas of healthcare.

Where things worked, it was because the health authority and locality commissioning group had a mature 'adult-to-adult' relationship and the health authority was happy to hand over the reins to commissioning groups as and when they were able or willing. A successful health authority was able to transfer appropriate and properly skilled staff to work with commissioning groups and the success of health authorities in the future will partly depend in the same way upon their willingness to devolve staff or management finance to their local PCGs.

Relating to trusts

Locality commissioning groups were particularly inventive in the way that they approached specialities, while trying to break down some of the barriers created at the time by trusts. Some formed strategy groups (such as the Northampton Commissioning Group) which allowed consultants from different trusts to meet with the GPs and co-operatively plan the way that local services were run. This meeting between GP and consultant, which was the basis of the relationship between many commissioning groups and trusts, was found to be extremely powerful. Discussing plans directly with consultants in the presence of health authority and trust managers made sure that any decisions were both workable and owned by both parties. The clinician-to-clinician interface also allowed GPs and consultants to look at restrictive practices on both sides, which were hampering progress but which could only be changed by one clinician speaking to another. The successful formula here was again mutual trust and respect, a desire to see things improve and acceptance that this should overcome factional interest. In many cases this proved to be more powerful than the contracting process itself, which became a rubber stamping exercise when the relationship between the trust and the commissioning group was sufficiently good.

That being said, the ability to move health authority contracts was an important bottom line when trusts were either not listening or refused to change. Long-term service agreements will act in the same way. Frequently, however, locality commissioning groups found themselves approached by managers, consultants and local trusts, who wished to introduce rational changes but required an 'outside authoritative' force to enable them to do so. This whole process of negotiating between GPs, specialists and managers involves a subtle mixture of diplomacy and perseverance but is undoubtedly one of the strongest forces for change that the NHS has ever seen. Peer review, as it were, with a difference!

Provision

Much of the work of PCGs will have more to do with provision than commissioning. Fund-holding showed that GPs could be successful at demand management in prescribing. Commissioning groups have looked at demand management in other areas such as orthopaedic operations (Mid Hampshire Commissioning Group) and it is becoming clear that what can be done for demand management and prescribing can also be done for diagnostics and referrals. Some examples have shown that the whole issue of using scarce resources cost-effectively is tied in with that of clinical governance. For instance, a con-certed effort to reduce unnecessary X-rays (e.g. Avon Commissioning Group) has saved money but also improved standards of care and patient health. Commissioning groups have shown a fast changing attitude toward peer review in localities where mutual trust has made doctors feel less vulnerable, more able to share information and acknowledge that they can improve their performance in various areas. The process demands a tactful and subtle approach, but within a safe environment it has often been the competitive element to improve on one's own performance (especially if others appear to be perform-ing far better) that has been a major key to improving standards by peer review. The experience has been that GPs are far too individualistic to accept peer review on any other terms.

Information

Commissioning needs good information and this will be an absolute requirement for the success of PCGs. Locality commissioning groups have valued the input from practices with sophisticated information technology, who have been able to double check or even produce new data at practice level for informing commissioning decisions. Historically, information systems have been far better in fundholding practices and their ability to share their systems and data with the commissioning group has led to a 'win/win' situation for both. Such arrangements will be important in future PCGs, although there is now a central realisation that there should be a fair upgrading of information systems within all practices.

Early wins

Early wins will be essential if PCGs are to gain the support and motivation of their members. When the PCG boards meet for the first time they are likely to find, just as locality commissioning groups did, that there are several areas where service provision is obviously poor and the answers are equally obvious. Several locality commissioning groups have, for instance, used 'yellow ticket' systems whereby problem areas are flagged up centrally on a day-to-day basis, and where areas are regularly underperforming they can be addressed by the group. Early wins will also be more achievable in the first days of a PCG because, just as locality commissioning groups found, health authorities and trusts will be eager to show their willingness to co-operate in the new process. There are many examples of early wins among commissioning groups[4] and these have included open access exercise ECG (Blackpool, Wyre and Fylde, Brent), a one-stop headache clinic (Dorset Commissioning Group) and NHS acute medical access to nursing homes (Huddersfield Commissioning Group). Some early wins have had little to do with commissioning groups and more to do simply with the spirit of co-operation between member practices such as the bulk purchasing of vaccines (Nottingham Commissioning Group), but these will also be relevant to PCGs. Words are fine but if a group can show real achievements to doubting health professionals and patients then its actions will speak louder than any words and provide the group with added momentum.

Conclusion

PCGs will be about relationships – efficient, productive relationships – and PCGs which are starting anew without any previous commissioning groups in the locality should perhaps find a local contact to discover the lessons that have been learnt. In his recent book *Effective Commissioning*,[7] Donald Light has argued that PCGs should not proceed to the upper 'options/levels' until they have achieved the social integration and sophistication of some of the more mature locality commissioning groups. There will be much emphasis on items such as the constitution of a PCG or the nature of its contracts with providers, but none of these things will fundamentally change our health system. They are essentially long stops, whose role is to police a system, which has failed in the first place because the relationships and motivation were not there to make it succeed. They have a role but it is secondary. What locality commissioning groups have shown PCGs, both in their mode of operation and their development, is just simply the old adage: 'Where there is a will there is a way'. If the motivation and the relationship is right then things will happen.

References

1 National Association of Commissioning GPs (1997) *Restoring the Vision.* National Association of Commissioning GPs, London.

2 Secretary of State for Health (1997) *The New NHS: modern, dependable.* Stationery Office, London.

3 NHS Primary Care Group Alliance website: *http://www.nhsalliance.org*

4 Dixon M, Murray T, Jenner D (1997) *The Locality Commissioning Handbook: from vision to reality.* Radcliffe Medical Press, Oxford.

5 Singer R (1997) *GP Commissioning: an inevitable evolution.* Radcliffe Medical Press, Oxford.

6   Singer R (1997) *GP Commissioning: an inevitable evolution*. Radcliffe Medical Press, Oxford, Chapter 3.

7   Light D (1998) *Effective Commissioning*. Office of Health Economics, London.

Further reading

Dixon M, Murray J, Jenner D (1997) *The Locality Commissioning Handbook: from vision to reality*. Radcliffe Medical Press, Oxford.

Light D (1998) *Effective Commissioning*. Office of Health Economics, London.

NHS Alliance Resource Pack (1998).

NHSE Resource Pack (1998).

Singer R (1997) *GP Commissioning: an inevitable evolution*. Radcliffe Press, Oxford.

Further information can be found on the NHS Alliance Website (*www.nhsalliance.org*).

PART 3

PCGs – back to the future

Peter Smith

The quest for organisational perfection has distracted many from the vexed question of how primary care groups (PCGs) will actually deliver better healthcare. Healthcare will not automatically be improved merely because we have groups of professionals and managers sitting around a table. Our 500 shiny new PCGs will quickly have to come to terms with their new functions. Many of these functions have already been developed within fundholding. Once the nature of the new PCGs is written indelibly in central guidance, the partisan fundholder/non-fundholder arguments become irrelevant. Atavistic antipathies should be forgotten – all are now working towards the same goal and all existing experience should be exploited to the full.

Fundholders already have extensive experience in many areas germane to PCGs, including prescribing, commissioning of secondary and community services, needs assessment, service review and primary care development. Most of these areas are dealt with elsewhere in this book, and have not been the exclusive domain of fundholders. Around the country, fundholders have successfully used fundholding as a tool to deliver value-added benefits. Most have become adept at innovating within tight constraints – the accountability framework of fundholding was far more stringent than that of PCGs. That expertise should be tapped by PCGs.

There is a wealth of experience from co-operative systems created despite the competitive nature of fundholding. Multifunds and total purchasing pilots (TPPs) in particular have already operated effectively as PCGs. For these groups, some aspects of PCGs are old news. However, the wider NHS changes offer the scope for greater innovation as the system places greater emphasis on true commissioning rather than currency and transactions.

The difference between mere purchasing and full commissioning can be illustrated by an analogy with the art world. If I attend an art exhibition I can buy what the exhibitors choose to present to me. It may be of good quality, but I am limited to what is on offer. If, however, I decide to *commission* a work of art I can choose the artist and even discuss with him or her the possible subject matter. The former is the old style of purchasing – there is some limited choice, but discussions will be based around price. The latter is the new style of commissioning – the emphasis is on the specification of the service within available resources. Many TPPs and multifunds have gained experience of this type of commissioning already. Most fundholders have strived to work towards this model. The following are some examples of the value-added innovations and principles of fundholding. Although specific schemes are quoted, every area will have similar developments. Those responsible for such developments should be seen as a resource for their PCG, not as ex-fundholders.

Identifying practice needs

If PCGs are to engage primary care, they will have to be seen to be addressing the needs of individual practices. Otherwise there will be no ownership from those delivering the service and the capacity to achieve change will be limited. Therefore always go for the bottom-up approach. Start with the practice needs and amalgamate these to establish the population needs. If PCGs are to deliver changes, this must happen within the practice. Each should complete a development plan, including how they would like services to change to meet the needs of their patients. These should then be amalgamated to form the basis of the service agreement, combined with activity and public health data. National priorities can then be used to strengthen relevant parts of the contract. The plans can be amalgamated to form the basis of the primary care investment plan.

The ability to combine primary care data obtained at practice level with secondary care data will eventually be a significant driver of the concept of integrated care. Until then, however, the practice is still the point at which the needs of the individual are fed into the system. For instance, practices with large numbers of nursing homes or residential homes for people with learning disabilities will be most aware of the needs of those populations. There will also be specific practices that will cover more deprived areas. Others will have GPs known to take an interest in certain conditions.

These aspects, among many others, will skew the needs of a population and will affect referrals, prescribing and staffing. Ultimately, it is the practice that will be best placed to effect change, but will need the support, resources and direction to help it achieve this. In-year problems will arise with specific 'expensive' patients who require justifiable extra resources. These will need to be provided without penalising the practice or the old perceived reluctance to take on 'expensive patients' will return.

A practice development plan need not be a complicated affair. Kingston and Richmond Multifund produced simple questionnaires and templates to assist practices in their decision making. Simple prompt sheets were also provided to encourage practices to consider new approaches to service delivery.

Tackling the giants: mental health, maternity and A&E

In the early stages most PCGs will want to tackle areas of local interest and achieve some quick successes. Since there is not the same annual round of contract negotiation, PCGs should consider beginning to look at bigger areas, out of the scope of traditional fundholding. To many these will be the most daunting area of PCG responsibility. Where primary care has become involved in these areas around the country, service developments have quickly followed. Multifunds and TPPs have addressed most major areas, including:

- A&E: Castlefields Surgery, Runcorn – monitored A&E attendances.
- Maternity: Berkshire Integrated Purchasing Pilot – implemented *Changing Childbirth*.
- Mental health and learning disabilities: Kingston and Richmond Multifund has developed service frameworks based on aggregate need and care planning rather than on face-to-face contacts.

Using high-quality management and administration

One of the most important lessons learnt by fundholders, multifunds and TPPs is that generally you will only be as successful as the abilities of the staff you employ allow. Many of the most successful fundholders did not have huge fundholding commitments. Their achievements relied on having very able staff to support them and run the fundholding system. Multifunds and TPPs developed sophisticated support structures to ensure that managers and technical staff, not primary care professionals, were responsible for the administrative workload. Staff previously employed within fundholding are a very valuable resource, and should be highly prized – they already have the experience in commissioning and primary care development so vital to PCGs.

Thus far, too little has been said about the support structures needed to run PCGs. They will need their own dedicated data managers, financial and accounts directors, and office teams. Healthcare professionals should not be expected to fulfil these roles except if they have made a decision to enter the field of management. It is obviously important that clinicians are involved in any stage where service changes are being discussed. Managers cannot be a substitute for clinical knowledge, as previous health authority commissioning proved. Most fundholders have learnt the hard way what can and what can't be delegated. PCGs should seek their advice or risk repeating the time-wasting mistakes of the previous systems. Examples of those who have experience of management issues include: any TPP or multifund, e.g. Kingston and Richmond Multifund, South West Thames Total Purchasing Pilot, Newham Inner City Multifund and Eastern Multifund, Belfast.

Contracting for quality

In the latter stages of fundholding, purchasing to achieve savings was replaced by contracting for quality. The contracting process was used as a tool to deliver quality improvements in secondary care. Using existing fundholder expertise, the same can rapidly be achieved within the new system across a PCG rather than for the benefit of a single practice.

Agreements with providers should be as robust as the previous 'contracts'. A rolling programme of three-year service agreements should allow us to escape the annual rush to reconfigure services matched by the annual attempts to resist it. Ideally we should now be able to develop services rationally within a sensible timescale.

What is particularly new about the latest form of service agreement is that it really is about defining a service, cutting across clinical directorate level. This finally allows for the possibility of formulating an agreement specifying inputs from different departments and clinical directorates.

Quality definition and monitoring will be crucial. With the loss of the annual intensive review, regular monitoring will be required to ensure adherence to the service agreement. Every agreement must include details of what is going to be monitored and how, with agreed limits, otherwise the agreement becomes a mere wish list and control over delivery of the service will be lost. For example, Castlefields Surgery in Runcorn, Cheshire made contracts specifying individual *consultants* and specific disease management pathways. Contracts were only made with consultants who agreed with the pathways, e.g. on grommets. Kingston and Richmond Multifund developed a core contract for services that specified realistic indicators of quality. Every paragraph includes an indication of what will be monitored and how.

Controlling out-of-area treatments (OATs)

At the time of writing it is far from clear what the 'currency' of the 'New NHS' is to be. One of the greatest benefits of the market was the understanding of where the money was really going. Fundholders have great experience in using resources effectively. This expertise will be at a premium as it becomes clear that some form of accounting system is again required to monitor activity against agreements and reign in the use of the potentially budget-blowing OATs. Around the country, fundholders have become used to weighing the arguments for and against potentially expensive, marginal treatments and conveying these to patients. This skill will have to be learnt by all PCG members. It will only take a couple of individual GPs sowing their wild OATs to decimate a budget.

All fundholders have extensive experience, along with their staff, of monitoring of ECRs. All have taken practice responsibility for them in different ways. Each PCG should speak to its local fundholders and ask them to show how they made the system work in their practices. Once again, it is the lesson of practice and GP level responsibility that needs to be learnt. Without it, PCGs will work much less effectively.

Good PR – making sure others know

It is vital that all the good work that is done is appreciated internally and externally. PCG boards have many levels of accountability – to their members, to the health authority and to the general public. Social services representatives on boards will have a responsibility to feed back and inform their own departments. Internal and external PR should be taken seriously. It is not just a case of spin doctoring. Details of negotiations, results and ongoing monitoring information should be fed back to users and members in a timely fashion. If not, trust will be lost and support will not be forthcoming when difficult decisions have to be made.

Many different methods have been used within fundholding to feed information back at a practice and corporate level. Many practices have used a fundholding notice board in the waiting room to keep the practice population informed about changes in contracting and what was being done for them. Despite the constant assertions to the contrary, most patients were unaware of whether their practice held a budget or not. Most will have a healthy disinterest in what most see as further NHS window dressing. What they are rightly interested in is what difference it makes to them.

Fundholding practices were required to produce regular reports which were public documents available to patients. Most multifunds produced annual reports detailing progress and financial summaries. These can be used to service a very wide audience. An example is the annual report produced by Kingston and Richmond Multifund, which was used at national, local, practice and GP level. The size of the document was always strictly controlled to make it readable and its emphasis was on important issues while still reminding the reader of the immense amount of background work required to make a multimillion pound organisation run effectively.

Time and again we hear that people should not receive information because they won't be able to understand it. Let's stop patronising the population – if they don't understand, it is our duty to explain it. Regular meetings of stakeholders should be held to allow feedback of important issues and open debate of important issues. Open PCG board meetings are unlikely to be the forum for debate. Although health authorities are required to have open board meetings, there is no requirement to allow observers to contribute.

This is only a brief overview of the lessons learnt by multifunds and TPPs. No PCG should feel they are heading into uncharted territory. The pioneers have been there before; it remains to be seen whether the path is now clear enough for others to follow. If in doubt, contact the groups referred to, your local fundholding practices, your nearest multifund or TPP. If you would like details of fundholders and fundholding groups (particularly TPPs and multifunds) who have pioneered changes, contact the National Association of Primary Care on 0171 636 1677.

CHAPTER THIRTEEN

How primary care commissioning can work: examples

Fran Butler

While the remit of primary care groups (PCGs) is much wider than that of total purchasing projects (TPPs) and GP commissioning groups, particularly with respect to primary care development and clinical governance, it is important that PCGs can learn from what has gone before. The purpose of this chapter is to describe a handful of initiatives undertaken by primary care-led commissioning groups over the past few years to demonstrate some of the reasonably 'quick hits' that could be achieved by PCGs.

There is an expectation that by working with each other, PCGs will make major strategic decisions, which will be incorporated in health improvement plans (HImPs); these decisions will affect the future direction of services and in some case the future of trusts. These will require consultation with and agreement of a large number of organisations and may take considerable time to implement. By contrast, the examples that follow are developments that could be made by single PCGs in collaboration with a small number of other organisations over a relatively short timescale. They have been set up fairly easily by the groups involved, but have enabled those within the groups to see that progress is being made and improvements for patients achieved.

Working with secondary care

This first example demonstrates primary care working with secondary care to set up an integrated service – in this case for back pain.

Developing a back pain service, Worth Valley Health Consortium and Airedale NHS Trust, Kevin Ellis, Contracting Contact

Setting

The Worth Valley Health Consortium is one of the first four TPPs and covers a population of 63 000 in Keighley, Haworth and Oakworth. It includes all seven practices and 37 GPs from the area, which covers an urban/rural mix, with pockets of high deprivation and a 6% Asian population. The consortium is the main purchaser of services from its local trust, Airedale NHS Trust.

The problem to be solved

Patients were experiencing long waits for physiotherapy and orthopaedic outpatient appointments. It was considered that there were inappropriate referrals to the orthopaedic consultants. There was no co-ordinated service for back pain sufferers and no anaesthesia-led back pain service.

The initiative

The consortium and the trust set out to develop a jointly agreed protocol for treating back pain. The aim was to improve secondary services for back pain, to shorten waiting times for physiotherapy and to provide an integrated pain relief service.

Achievements

Joint guidelines were agreed covering primary and secondary treatment of back pain, and a joint back pain clinic was established at Airedale, consisting of a senior physiotherapist, rheumatologist and an orthopaedic surgeon specialising in backs. Additional resources were put into community physiotherapy and working practices were rearranged to enable patients to be assessed within two weeks. A pain relief service was purchased from the private sector and some joint injections were purchased from primary care.

Patient feedback was extremely encouraging, being positive about both the short waits and their speed of treatment.

Problems experienced

Concerns were initially expressed about the back pain service being swamped with referrals. It was therefore decided that it would be appropriate for most of the referrals to come from physiotherapists, and only if the GP was sure of the diagnosis was he or she to refer directly to the back pain clinic. This led to few referrals directly from GPs.

Additionally, because no pain relief service was available at Airedale, it had to be offered at a different centre and GPs tended to refer directly to this rather than to the back pain clinic.

What we would do differently

Better communication with physiotherapists on the ground would ensure appropriate referrals. We would also integrate the pain relief service into the back pain clinic, including the psychological input as well as physical help.

What are the next steps?

We would like Airedale to offer the integrated pain relief at back pain clinics as described above. We also intend to expand primary care facilities and increase the number of joint injections where appropriate.

Relevance for PCGs

This type of partnership working, using established best practice and agreeing joint protocols to develop a care pathway including primary and secondary input, is a model for future development of integrated patient-focused services.

Improving links with the community

In this example a GP commissioning pilot demonstrates how practices working with community development representatives can achieve a more integrated approach to community development.

Health and Community Liaison Group, Dunstable & Houghton Regis Commissioning Pilot, Elaine Richardson, Project Manager

Setting

The commissioning pilot involves 12 practices covering 75 000 population. It is located primarily in the urban areas of Dunstable and Houghton Regis and the villages of Caddington and Toddington.

The problem to be solved

The pilot identified the development of links with key stakeholders in community development in South Bedfordshire as a key step to achieving a more integrated approach to the production and implementation of health alliance and community care. A South Bedfordshire Community Care Development Group (SBCCDG) was convened to develop the more integrated approach at a strategic level.

The initiative

The Health and Community Liaison Group arose out of a chance conversation between a local authority and health authority manager after a SBCCDG meeting. The group initially focused on one particular geographical area where resources were already being invested in community development, the aim being to develop links between local authority officers and general practices with a view to identifying opportunities for joint working.

The decisions to keep the group small and the aim relatively loose were deliberate, as the starting point was virtually zero. An initial meeting involving the local authority manager, her leisure centre manager, the community development officer, the health authority manager and two practice managers enabled people to start to understand the scope of local authority and general practice involvement in the area. Following a brainstorming session on potential areas for joint working, the development of a resource file was immediately identified as an opportunity to take forward. This file would contain details of local groups, facilities and activities and a copy would be held at the practices so that patients could be advised of what was available. Leaflets about local authority initiatives, such as holiday clubs and exercise promotions, are also now regularly sent to practices.

The group felt there was real benefit in continuing to meet not only to develop particular projects and share information but also to learn more about what each member does. It was recognised that as there was no specific funding for the group most projects would need to utilise existing resources, so small projects were more likely to be successful.

Achievements

Achievements so far include:

- A community notice board displaying information about local facilities and activities has been set up in the waiting room of one of the practices. The same practice is working with the community arts officer to provide a wall on which a local group can produce a mural and use the practice in the 'Gallery on Wheels' project.
- Exchange visits have been set up between the practices and leisure centres and an initiative on promoting exercise with patients has commenced.
- Practice managers are attending local practitioners groups.
- A project looking at how baby clinics can be used to promote play and parenting skills has been initiated.

The group has grown to include another area of deprivation and, while no formal evaluation has taken place, this expansion demonstrates the fact that the individuals involved see a benefit in the approach. The aim of the group has clearly been achieved, as the practice managers not only have an increased understanding of community development but are also getting actively involved. Likewise local authority officers have a much clearer understanding of the constraints and opportunities in general practice. The major disadvantage is that the group's success is dependent on the interest and enthusiasm of those involved.

Relevance for PCGs

PCGs need to work in partnership with local authorities and the type of approach above supports working at an operational level even though a different approach may be needed at a strategic one.

Evidence-based healthcare

Practices in a consortium of fundholding practices have worked together to develop and introduce evidence-based protocols to ensure their patients receive effective preventative care.

Secondary prevention of ischaemic heart disease, West Berkshire Fundholding Consortium, Dr Nigel McFetridge, GP, Brookside Group Practice

Setting

The West Berkshire Fundholding Consortium is a group of ten fundholding practices, which agreed to work together on a variety of commissioning issues. The practices cover about 100 000 patients across rural and urban areas.

Problem

In 1996, the practices agreed that the next step in the development of fundholding should be to focus on areas where there was strong evidence of effectiveness of interventions or services, particularly where they resulted in overall health gain. Secondary prevention of heart disease was chosen.

The initiative

The work started with a literature review of the current evidence of effectiveness of the various possible interventions and an assessment of their possible cost implications. A steering group was then set up to address issues of implementation.

The objective was that the ten WBFC practices and demonstrate that all their patients who have a history of heart attack or angina are receiving the most effective programme of preventative care within the resources available. This required that each practice identified those patients registered with them who had a history of myocardial infarction or angina and then reviewed their current lifestyle and medication to minimise their risk of further coronary events. A set of guidance notes that included a suggested protocol was distributed to all the practices. Briefly, patients were stratified into four groups of descending risk of a further coronary event. Starting with highest risk group first, patients were asked to complete a questionnaire and to attend a 10-minute lifestyle advice consultation with the practice nurse. The nurse focused on the most important lifestyle issue raised in the questionnaire. An appointment was then made for the patient to see their doctor who reviewed their prevention therapy.

Key features of the initiative

The evidence-based medicine approach has to mix science with pragmatism. There are many gaps in the evidence. For example, do we restrict prescribing only to the statins demonstrated to improve overall outcome, or do we prescribe the statin which is cheapest but possibly not fully researched?

Best practice may not be attainable within available resources. Most guidelines promote best practice. The key (unique?) feature of this project was the development of guidelines promoting best practice within unpredictable available resources.

Evidence is increasing that lifestyle changes have at least the same benefit on outcome as some drug interventions, e.g. a high intake of oily fish, garlic (especially raw!), nuts and vitamin E. So in the project, equal weight was given to lifestyle interventions as to drug interventions.

Achievements

The practices have adopted the approach to varying degrees and all are involved in secondary prevention of ischaemic heart disease. While the impact has not been formally evaluated, many lessons have been learned which are particularly relevant to the emerging PCGs and HImPs.

Problems

Adopting a multidisciplinary approach is very difficult in a changing environment of staff, knowledge, views of best practice and organisational relationships. But many factors were not a problem: motivation, bringing together relevant knowledge, skills and experience, and being explicit about prioritisation.

However, other factors were a problem: getting time for training, not having the time to provide a comprehensive service, lack of national guidance, gaps in the evidence, staff leaving and variation in practice information systems.

Next steps and relevance to PCGs

This project set out to take a multidisciplinary approach to implementing evidence-based practice by focusing on outcomes that result in health gain at a community level. This approach is now at the heart of PCG function and HImPs. It is hoped that this project will form the starting point of the development of a 'health improvement toolkit' and work has started on this.

Moving care closer to the community and avoiding delayed discharge

The next example is from the New River Total Care Project, a TPP. The project demonstrates liaison between practices and secondary care to facilitate discharge and reduce length of stay, and the provision of more appropriate settings for patients not requiring acute support.

Community liaison team, New River Total Care Project, Liz Wise, Project Manager

Setting

The New River Total Care Project is a second wave TPP involving five practices and a total of 58 000 patients in north London. Two of the practices are located within the Tomlinson area and two have a higher than average population of elderly patients on their list.

The problem to be solved

The problem we initially sought to address was one of information and liaison. GPs frequently were unaware of the admission of their patients to hospital or of the timing or quality of their discharge. In addition, they wished to ensure appropriateness of care for their patients and to maximise the use of 'step-down' rehabilitative GP beds in Enfield Community Care Centre. The initial remit of the team was therefore to maintain records of the project's patients in local hospitals and keep the GP practices informed of this, to facilitate discharge, ensuring safety and appropriateness, and to arrange transfer of patients to the GP unit once their acute phase was over.

The initiative

The project's community liaison team consists of two and a half whole-time equivalent nurses, attached to the practices within the project, together with an administrative officer. The team is employed by the local community care trust.

Originally named the discharge liaison team, the community liaison team developed over the past two and a half years beyond its original remit to facilitate patients' discharge and track and provide information to the GPs on their patients in hospital.

After its first year the team extended its remit and function to include community liaison, hence the change of name. The team felt that the existing discharge processes were robust and that some duplication was occurring. They now become involved in only complex discharges where some facilitation and liaison are required, but have extended their role to prevent admissions and work with vulnerable elderly patients. In addition to providing information on admissions and discharges to the practices, the team now also follows up through direct patient contact, either visiting or by telephone, all over-75-year-olds who attend local A&E departments, with a view to identifying unmet needs which could prejudice health and result in readmission. The team also follows up discharge patients with multifaceted needs with a similar purpose.

Formal evaluation is currently underway, carried out by the public health department of Enfield and Haringey Health Authority. This includes a survey of other healthcare professionals who have indicated their clear support for the service. Other indicators under review are readmission rates, delayed discharge rates and estimates of bed days saved. The team's view, however, is that the scheme has overwhelming intangible benefits as well. The nurses are now a resource to community and hospital as well as carers and patients, in terms of their knowledge of local health and social services and how to access them. The effect of such a service on the long-term health of patients is more difficult to estimate.

Problems experienced

The main problems encountered arose in the financial arena. The Total Care Project was born in a time of extreme financial pressure for the health authority and had no access to development or growth funds. Its development was therefore of necessity self-financing, with, to put it crudely, bed days saved and admissions prevented funding the service. While our community trust was willing to contract with the project on an occupied bed day basis, allowing the release of moneys (albeit at marginal rates) to fund this service, the acute trusts felt unable to do this. This is because despite reducing patients' length of stays the costs remained the same, in some cases higher if step-down care was accessed. This undoubtedly influenced the direction of the team's work away from acute care.

Relevance to PCGs

As PCGs are formed, the project's GPs are looking to widen such an initiative across the PCGs. The practice-attached nature of this service lends itself to development in this way, although funding will be an issue, as savings are unlikely to be realised at the level required in the initial phases. The local acceptance and popularity of the scheme with GPs are likely to make this a priority for the future.

Working with other agencies

In the following examples, a TPP which is now a shadow PCG has worked with other agencies, including voluntary groups, to address some of the causes of ill health. PCGs have a principle function of improving the health of the population. The examples listed below are about health, rather than healthcare, and have increased the awareness of GPs and other members of the primary healthcare trust of the wider determinants of health.

Working with other agencies, Daventry and South Northamptonshire Primary Care Alliance (DPA), Shaun Brogan, Chief Executive, DPA

Introduction

Three initiatives from DPA are described below, all of which involve working with agencies outside the health service.

Setting

DPA is a total purchasing project which grew, in stages, into an embryo PCG. It now consists of 12 practices, covering a population of 93 000 and about 60 GPs. The PCG covers most of Daventry and South Northamptonshire Council areas, with a predominantly rural population. There is no gross deprivation, although many in the area express concern about hidden rural deprivation.

Carers referral project

The problem to be solved

There was felt to be a lack of care and concern for carers with the project. Carers represent an unsung and unrewarded 'asset' of the NHS because they look after people who would otherwise fall to the care of the health service or social services. This would cost large sums of money. It is often said that if all carers ceased to care for their relative(s) or friend(s) tomorrow, the cost to the state of looking after all these additional people would be billions of pounds.

The initiative

The aim of the initiative is to provide advice and help for carers who themselves need care. Members of the primary care team (GPs, nurses, therapists, etc.) would identify any carers whom they believe need care and attention themselves and refer these carers to a carers' support clinic run at DPA (as part of a range of outpatient clinics). All members of the primary care team have been given copies of a yellow carers' referral card. This enables them to refer carers to the carers' advice clinic at DPA. The clinic runs once a month.

Achievements and problems experienced

Carers have been referred by primary care team members to the carers' clinic. However, although the clinic has been running for over a year, fewer than expected carers have been referred. The question is being asked whether all the carers in the area who themselves need care and attention have in fact been referred, or whether some are being 'missed' (perhaps because the primary care team members are focusing too much on the ill or disabled person the carer is looking after).

Next steps

DPA is discussing with the Northamptonshire Carers' Association ways in which the numbers of referrals can be increased.

Benefits advice referrals project

The problem to be solved

The poverty and resulting ill health arising from the poor take-up of benefits.

The initiative

The aim of this initiative is to increase the take-up of benefits among those eligible to receive them, thereby alleviating poverty and inequality to some extent, with the ultimate aim of improving the health of these people.

All the members of the primary care team have been given copies of a green benefits referral card. This enables them to refer people in need to Daventry Welfare Rights or the citizens' advice bureau.

Achievements and problems experienced

Daventry Welfare Rights and the citizens' advice bureau both report a substantial increase in benefits 'referrals'. The project has now added a tick box to the green card to try to ascertain how many referrals are originating with primary healthcare team members. Very few problems have been experienced.

Next steps

One of the DPA practices is now collaborating with Daventry Welfare Rights and the citizens' advice bureau to identify all people over 65 years on their computer. All these people will then be offered a benefits check. This particular practice carried out this exercise a few years ago and the result was a substantial increase in benefit take-up. If this exercise is similarly successful we will work to persuade all DPA practices to carry out the same exercise.

Young persons' sexual health clinic

The initiative

The aims of this project are:

- to reduce teenage pregnancies
- to address the anxieties that young people have about sex, contraception, relationships and drugs.

The objective of the project is to ally with a well-respected local voluntary group 'Time to Talk' (T2T) to provide sexual health clinics as one part of their range of advice and other services for young people.

A DPA GP and practice nurse run a regular clinic in the T2T premises. The health authority funds T2T to provide a variety of services for young people. With health authority encouragement and support, T2T now 'purchases' the services of the DPA GP and nurse that run this clinic.

Achievements and problems experienced

There has been a slow but steady increase in visits to this clinic. T2T and DPA are extremely pleased with the success of this initiative. Very few problems have been encountered.

Next steps

T2T and DPA are now planning to open a new clinic in the south of the DPA area (in Towcester) to serve young people in that area.

Index